The Red of My Blood

www.penguin.co.uk

Also by Clover Stroud

The Wild Other
My Wild and Sleepless Nights

The Red of My Blood

A Death and Life Story

Clover Stroud

doubleday

TRANSWORLD PUBLISHERS
Penguin Random House, One Embassy Gardens,
8 Viaduct Gardens, London SW11 7BW
www.penguin.co.uk

Transworld is part of the Penguin Random House group of companies
whose addresses can be found at global.penguinrandomhouse.com

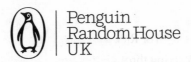

First published in Great Britain in 2022 by Doubleday
an imprint of Transworld Publishers

This is a work of non-fiction based on the life, experiences and
recollections of the author. In some limited cases names of people
and places have been changed to protect the privacy of others.

A CIP catalogue record for this book
is available from the British Library.

ISBN 9780857527738

Typeset in 10.25/16pt Optima LT Pro by Jouve (UK), Milton Keynes
Printed and bound in Great Britain by Clays Ltd, Elcograf S.p.A.

The authorized representative in the EEA is Penguin Random House Ireland,
Morrison Chambers, 32 Nassau Street, Dublin D02 YH68.

Penguin Random House is committed to a sustainable future
for our business, our readers and our planet. This book is made
from Forest Stewardship Council® certified paper.

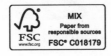

For Rick and Alexandra.
Walking through this time beside you
has shown me we are Argonauts,
we are astronauts, we are deep-sea divers.

Prologue

In October 2015 my sister was diagnosed with stage 4 breast cancer. She was given chemotherapy and radiotherapy, but after being given the all-clear in 2016, she developed breast cancer again. She had more treatment, but after clear scans in 2017, the following year she learned the cancer had metastasized and spread to her bones. She continued to have treatment throughout 2019, and by November, despite her secondary diagnoses, her oncologist was cautiously optimistic about her future. He hoped she'd have at least another five, possibly even ten more years. Ten days later, in early December 2019 she was admitted to hospital with a suspected small blood clot on her lung. She was expected to stay in for a week. 'Don't worry, Clo, I'm going to pull through this,' she said to me on the telephone from hospital on 6 December. 'We're going to have lots more adventures together.'

On 7 December 2019, her blood results showed she had advanced liver failure. She died at 4.20 p.m. on 8 December 2019. She was two years older than me and forty-six years old.

Chapter 1

Dark Rooks

Words. So many words to deal with in the days after death. Many of them were senseless to me. Sometimes they would seem to materialize from nowhere. Suddenly I would hear a voice: 'Mind yourself, there's a van, the lights haven't changed yet.' A woman's voice, her hand touching my arm, to stop me stepping out in front of traffic on a kerbside in Oxford. I was walking through a city I'd known all my life, but I was entirely lost.

'Can I get you anything else? Would you like anything else?' I thought I knew what the woman behind the shop till meant, but I couldn't make sense of the sounds coming from her mouth.

'If you do decide on a burial in a portion of the land where she lived, you will need to find out if a watercourse runs through it. It's certainly complicated burying someone on private land, but not impossible.'

That was at the undertaker's, three days later, where I had gone to make plans. We were discussing an idea, and this one was that my dead sister might be buried in the field she owned beside her house. I was finding it easier to concentrate on the colours around him than on the words he said. They were a simpler place to exist within than the words he said to me, which landed in my head like dark rooks. These colours were better things to think about than his words: his black suit with a royal blue tie and the brown mahogany polished table in his office with its red curtains, the yellow roses, possibly synthetic, in a golden jug with a black pattern around it that looked Greek. And the tight, reassuring buttons of the red velvet chesterfield where I sat as we talked about the arrangements for her funeral. They were the only things I could make out that felt real and physical. My sister must be in a refrigerator somewhere in this building, I realized, as I ran my hands between the buttons, concentrating on them and pressing the tips of my fingers into the indentations in the red velvet where the buttons sat. I forced my thumbs into the material so that I could feel my body, and when I did that, I noticed that the ends of my thumbs went very red too, although my hands looked quite pale. And it was easier to concentrate on the shiny red velvet since it was too unbearable to think about either the watercourse which might run across her coffin buried deep underground, making her body disintegrate faster, or the shape of the refrigerator she was lying in, although that was the thing my brain kept circling back to. I wondered how cold it was inside that refrigerator. What temperature was the refrigerator she lay in? How long was it? How wide was it? Could I have fitted beside it if I lay down with her? How long could I have lain there stretched beside her?

Also, the golden jug with the geometric Greek pattern. As I thought about the refrigerator, I realized the golden jug was then the only thing I could see in the room.

I had tried to put make-up on before going to the undertaker's. Mascara and eyeliner normally make me feel like a more clearly defined version of myself, and I needed this definition since I was aware I might be vanishing. Most of the time I moved slowly around the house with my shoulders hunched; if you had seen me, you might have thought I was sick. I moved like someone with an acute illness and had the outline of a very old person. A lot of the time I did not hear or could not properly make out the voices of other people talking around me, not even the voices of my husband Pete and my children, Jimmy and Dolly, who were nineteen and sixteen at that time, and Evangeline, Dash and Lester, who were seven, five and three. When someone dies, there are so many voices and you don't know who they belong to or how to identify them. Sometimes you don't care who they belong to because what does it matter if the car insurance that's in arrears is cancelled, as the voice on the phone reminds you, or the back pain from that slipped disc you thought was so bad a week ago – before she died or was anywhere close to dying – does actually put you into a wheelchair, which is what the chiropractor you know quite well says will happen if you don't do the Pilates she is always talking about? Her life is over, so you feel as if your life is over too. In fact, you want your life to be over. You would welcome it. Mostly, the only voice you are listening out for is that of the one person you most certainly could identify, but which you now cannot hear anywhere. You are worrying what it might feel like to lose the memory of the sound of that voice amongst the noise. You wonder if it is possible to preserve the sound of the voice of the dead person in your head forever. You think of the many, many, many things you should have said to her, all through your lives together, to be completely sure, utterly sure, that she knew how much you loved her. If you really ask yourself the truth, you know she knew. But you still wish you had the chance for that conversation one more time. So all the other voices around you mean nothing.

Even my children shouting at me and one another, later that night, after I got back from the undertaker's, did not mean anything. I could not hear their demands. In the bathroom, I knelt on the wooden floor as the room filled with steam and condensation, the sound of the water falling from the tap into the bath so loud that I could barely hear my two young sons yelling about who would slide down the slippery side of the bath into it first. One of them was screaming so loudly that I couldn't think but I wondered why a small child aged three would choose to shriek like that, as if he was shouting at the existence of life itself.

I pulled T-shirts from their fuzzy blond heads, unbuttoned their little jeans, crouching down to pull them off, noticing that they were both getting too big for their clothes, and as I knelt at their feet, I thought of Christ kneeling before his disciples and I wondered if he knew how and when he would die. He knew he was going to die; we all know we are going to die. And then, also, I wondered if I was now in a world of death quite separate from Jesus, but more like the Old Testament. It felt like that inside my head. My sister and I had been through a lot of intense experiences which had in a way taken us close to death together, and certainly right inside a trauma that we both had lived with all the time. In the bathroom with my sons shouting at one another, I thought back to my last experiences of life and death, so recent, lying beside her in her hospital bed. I had held her extremely close. I'd been able to smell her skin and the frankincense my stepmother dropped on to her pale cotton shirt because my sister loved that smell. I had squeezed her. I had thought that I could maybe squeeze through the portal with her if I held on to her tightly enough. 'Cling on, cling on,' we used to say to each other sometimes when we were hugging one another, especially in late adolescence and our early twenties when the imprint of adult life lay more softly on us, before trauma imprinted itself there. It was what I wanted to do in those last hours of her life. Cling on, cling on, so that I could go with her and would not actually find myself here, kneeling beside a running bath, separated from her in her death and forever.

I had also very much wanted to ask her what it felt like to be dying. On her last day, she knew she was dying. One day, said the consultant with the serious voice (it couldn't really have been anything else, could it?) as he knelt down beside her bed and told her she was dying. Because she was a warrior. She wanted the truth so she could go on to the next field equipped and ready.

'A day,' she said to my father, looking up at him as he stood, beloved, at her bedside when he arrived at the hospital.

'I have a day to live.'

I wanted to know what it would feel like to know there was only a day left; I wonder if it gave you a shooting-into-another-universe feeling, as if you could inhabit an entire lifetime in twenty-four hours. I think, though I am not completely certain, that this is what I saw my sister doing in that one day she had left. She lived everything in that day while looking directly into the face of death and knowing she was going there. As my sister lay dying, I wanted to ask her what she was feeling so that I could feel it with her too and become a part of it with her. I wanted to ask her: what is happening? Does this feel the same as the other things we have been through together – when we talked about Mum and what happened to her – or is this quite different? Where are you now? Can you smell the drops of frankincense on your shirt and are you here or somewhere else? What can you see? Are you afraid or do you feel joy or is this a relief? What does this feel like?

This was what I thought about, now that she was dead and I was kneeling in the bathroom before my children, pulling their trousers from them, feeling as though I was part of the Bible – Old or New Testament, I still wasn't sure.

Golden orange was the colour I saw most often in the days that followed her death. Each day I was walking through deep emotion, but colours could be signs of messages to watch for when words were inadequate and those emotions overwhelmed me. And because it was Christmas time, there was golden orange everywhere: in the tinsel wrapped around a green plastic tree beside the receptionist's office in school; in the twists of foiled paper covering sweets Dash and Evangeline came home with; in the delicate tissue paper of the crowns that fell out of crackers, snapped unseasonably early since that year wasn't like Christmas at all. A lot of people brought presents over to the house for the children, from 9 December onwards, the day after my sister's death, and although I looked at them and was not really sure what they were for (had the well-wrapped objects been brought to the house early by kind, sad people as a sort of consolation for the fact my sister had died?), the children loved this. Without me nearby to control them they ripped through the piles in the sitting room, leaving wrapping paper and toys and books scattered around. They also pulled the boxes of crackers with each other, even though I had thought I had hidden them so well in the back of a cupboard in my bedroom. I'd bought the crackers in a charity shop in November, but when I'd done so I couldn't have seen what was coming on 8 December, since at that point death wasn't close to our lives. I didn't mind the children opening all the presents early. Presents opened weeks before Christmas Day didn't mean anything. I didn't mind them pulling the crackers they'd uncovered either. Crackers snapped before school didn't matter. The children ate marshmallows and chocolate and the cake for breakfast that the sad, thoughtful people brought to the house, and the ends of crackers piled up in the wastepaper basket in the bathroom. But this didn't matter. Nothing mattered. Except that she was dead and we needed to organize her funeral.

The other colour was petrol blue, that beautiful, strange colour you see on some birds' wings if you ever get near enough to them. Mostly, rooks, ravens and crows just look like big black birds, but if you see one close up, so close that you can actually touch a wing and lay the feathers on it flat, there is another shade there too: a petrol-blue colour that's very deep and only visible in certain light, so it's kind of magical and strange. But you don't see it often, as I say. Now, though, I was aware of being very close to that colour all the time. Being in the hospital as my sister breathed for the last time had given me the sense that I was walking around with another being very, very close to me, close enough to see its strange powerful colours. And this was death.

My mascara stopped helping me feel like myself. It poured down my face in black lines as soon as I applied it. I stood in front of the mirror and imagined pencilling big black panda rings around my eyes and bright red clown lips and thick brushes of peach-pink blusher across my cheeks to colour myself into existence. Most of the time I felt as if I was seeping into nothing. I was diluting as she left me.

My mind needed strong, solid things for it to hold on to so I thought of the stone knights with their swords beside them who lay so still in their cold beds in Gloucester Cathedral. She had been like one of them when she died, still and strong and eternal, or a Pharaoh, magnificent and golden. I have seen two other dead people in my life but I have never before seen a golden dead person. She was golden. I am not lying about that or imagining it. I took a photo of her when she was dead and I look at it sometimes if I am feeling entirely strong or exceptionally reckless and I can tell you, she was golden. She was like a god.

I'd felt extremely weird taking that photo. Mostly, we photograph happy holidays and big family meals, posing with cocktails. Or we record children on bicycles or splashing on the beach or eating picnics by a river or the new paint job in the sitting room. We capture the bright and gleaming moments. We do not photograph death. Also, my sister had just died. I was in the room with my dead sister. It felt completely inappropriate to be photo-graphing her. But now I can see my golden sister inside my phone whenever I want and I am happy I have that photograph.

Four days after she had died, I found myself lying in bed making the same shape she had made in those last two days of her life in hospital. I lay stone still in a way I have never done before. I wondered if I was adopting the position of death. I wondered whether, if I got closer to death, I could be closer to her. When I spoke, I felt as if my voice did not sound like my own. It was deeper, more like her deep voice. I felt as though part of her had entered into me when she died. I knew that I had the same DNA as her so a part of her *was* me. I also knew that my body and marrow and blood and bones and the emotional life we had lived through together, especially our time as adolescents in the years after Mum's accident, meant that, apart from our seven children, we were closer to each other than anyone else alive. I hoped death could slide over me and show me that still, golden serenity it had shown her. Maybe I could turn into a god too. But then I realized that the afternoon was turning to dusk and that it was getting cold and I needed to turn the lamp on in my bedroom, so I sat up. And the way I was crying made me cough and then choke, and I swore and realized I was in no way close to death. I was revoltingly alive and human, sweating despite the cold, and weeping, snotty, my hair greasy, much too alive.

In those first days immediately after her death, whenever I was in the kitchen the demands of physical and mortal life overwhelmed me. I could concentrate on her funeral because that was a ceremony with poetry and song and incense so it was the ritual I could hang my sorrow on. I hoped domestic life might be at least small and manageable after having been in the massive presence of death, but in fact I found emptying the dishwasher or listening to Evangeline's spelling practice disorientated me. It sent my brain skittering like marbles, so that I lost pieces of it under the sofa as my thoughts gathered with the lint and sweet wrappers stuck in the edge of the black and pink rug stretched out across the wooden floor. I kept trying to gather myself because although the colour all around me now was the petrol blue of rooks' wings, as I told you, pieces of my life still needed attending to. I needed to cook things or undress the children or speak to my father on the telephone. But when I was in the house with Pete and the children – and not at that undertaker's, for example, or outside the house doing things like driving to pick up certificates or view burial plots – I felt separate and alone. When I looked at my children, I thought of the pain they would one day feel when they lost one of their siblings. I fervently prayed I too would be dead by then, but that scared me too, since it meant I would not be there to comfort the living siblings. I petrified myself thinking about the agony that lay before them in their lives, which was an absolutely irrefutable fact. If I could have turned myself to stone at this point to avoid thinking of the pain I would have done. I thought of all the living my children had gone through together and it made me think of all the living I had gone through with my sister and I could not fathom how the constant of our forty-four and a half years together as sisters had now finished and was over. My children were hurting, but it was different. Sometimes they looked at me with bruised red faces, or suddenly burst into tears when they were brushing their teeth, but she was their aunt. She was my sister. An entire lifetime shared. A childhood lived always at each other's side, twin beds in a room lined with toy monkeys, an adolescence stumbled through, trauma and loss navigated together while it shaped us into everything that we were, adult life forged with the force of blacksmiths hammering metal. And now it was over? Now I was expected to keep on living without her? Yes, death had taken that from me, and no one alive would ever be that to me again. So I was right to feel alone. I was alone. And I felt as if I had drunk hemlock, secretly, so that I was the only one in the kitchen who had been poisoned. Pete and the children certainly felt very sad, but I felt distanced from them by the mortal poison that was now running through my being.

And yet, I felt like them. I felt like a child. Sometimes I needed to be told what to do, which clothes to wear, how to walk into and out of the day. Sometimes I wasn't completely sure I knew how to walk, or swallow, or breathe. Everything that I feared about loss and the way it had been with me and part of me every single day since I was sixteen when Mum's accident had left her with brain damage so bad she never spoke again was true once more, because now my sister was gone too and so loss was everywhere and on everything. Other people came into the house on those days. I took the children to school but in the days straight after death a friend picked them up. I didn't know at the time where I was but I knew I wanted to be close to my father and my stepmother.

Somehow, I knew who I was when I was with them. At other times I felt other people – friends, a mother from school – putting a plate of food in front of me.

'Here, eat. Take this and eat it,' I heard someone say while I was sitting at the kitchen table as my brain spun, but the food tasted of nothing and I could not tell you what it was or who had made it either.

It was much, much better when no one asked me how I was, but people did ask me this. 'How *are* you?' they would say, maybe someone who had arrived at the house to drop off a meal or deliver back one of the children's book bags left at school. They meant well, but oh my God how can you answer that question? What words can you use to answer that? Language was failing me all over the place. I look back at my notebooks of the time and I have written almost nothing but 'I feel sad' many times over. If I had been able to express myself more clearly, I might have said something Gilgamesh said: 'Death lives in the house where my bed is and wherever I set my feet, there Death is.'

I did not have the capacity to make words perform for me like this when I said them aloud. In my head, though, words did still work. In my head, my voice spoke to me all the time, even when I was talking to someone else. In my head, there were always words going around, asking me, their owner, to explain what had been happening and how this could have happened, and who I should find to tell me what to feel, think, say, do and most of all locate *where,*

where, where she had gone. Also, words worked for me when I was driving, since I was not so confused that I could not get in the car; and they worked for me, too, when lying on the sofa in Dash and Lester's room, reading to them.

I could not have read books about wizards or trains or ponies since sweet and funny childish things like that didn't seem to have a place in my life any more. (At the children's nativity play, four days after my sister's death, I watched Dash, Lester and Evangeline with little mouths like red Os singing about an angel appearing on a hill with a halo bright, and my shoulders shook as I cried, so that I was ashamed I would be disturbing the family in the plastic seats behind me.) I would have liked to read the Bible, because the words in it are so old that they are consoling, whatever truth or not you locate in them, or some ancient poetry, but if I'd done that my small sons might have started shouting at me. Instead, I read, for as long as twenty minutes at a time, from a book called *Arthur and His Knights of the Round Table*, by Roger Lancelyn Green, because we all liked the stories in this.

There was something eternal, and also brave (which is important), within the tales of knights who left the court for difficult adventures. It's not that the knights were not afraid of what lay ahead, but they confronted their fear straight on, like Gawain facing the Green Knight. What they went in search of often wasn't what they returned with, and mostly they went alone. Lying in the boys' room on the sofa with the ripped covers where my children had pulled out the stuffing, I felt safer and more secure than I did in the rest of my life. Knowing that these knights faced the darkest part of the forest – where the frost lay undisturbed, since their path was one they walked alone, riding into the densest brambles, where the thorns were sharpest and the red of the wild roses most vivid – was reassuring, because that made me feel I could do it too.

It was as if the knights had always been out on those journeys into the dark forest, and by reading about them I sensed that they might be able to show me something or help me find something that had utterly gone from my life. When I thought about them, I felt less alone. Or perhaps not less alone, but that there might be a path in this forest for me to find too.

The children liked the stories, even when they became quite complicated, but what I liked best was the names dropping on to the page: Arthur Pendragon, Galahad, Lancelot, Gawain. They were names that spoke of a bravery I could believe in. They were also people doing something very active. They were not confused or lost or broken or felled, and even if they felt those things, their sense of their quest still took them forwards. As a result, the knights *knew what to do* in the face of adversity, hardship and challenge.

And also they just sounded extremely ancient, and that was comforting, and kind of beautiful, since the present moment was such an uncomfortable place to be and nothing in it reassured me or even seemed solid. At times I wondered if the present moment actually existed at all.

*

Five days after she died, I walked out on to the cold wet ground in the field near the house because there was something like a salve in the sharpness of the air and the smell of green earth around me. Every part of me felt drenched and sodden with sadness and pain, and I thought that moving, outside, might feel like lancing a wound: relief. I wanted to take myself to a place where I might find my sister, and also a place where I could feel brave.

Horses represent something ancient and heroic to me, so I went outside into the wet winter air because standing at the gate of the field near our house was the horse I had had for some time. I'd sent my sister a picture of myself on this horse two months before and she had messaged me back *WOW*. I tried not to think of where her *WOW* wonder had gone or allow into my head the idea that I'd never ride with her ever again or the thought of her now lying in a refrigerator, but instead I put my arms around the neck of that horse. I saw myself reflected in the mare's eye, and when I pressed my face into her mane, black and white because she was a Gypsy horse, my breath was full and deep, not shallow and failing as it had felt for days, and there was other relief in that.

Her silver shoes glinted through the mud as I led her from the field, and in the careful way she placed her huge hooves, as big as plates, I felt she was minding my feet too. Her saddle and her bridle smelt good when I cinched the buckles, of clean leather, and for a few moments I felt competent because this act proved I could do something. I know about horses and have always had them in my life so tacking her up was automatic. It wasn't difficult. Plates might slip from my hands and smash on the kitchen floor when I approached the dishwasher, but I could saddle up my horse.

It had been raining, and the ground under her hooves squelched, the only sound apart from the leather of her saddle squeaking and the chink of her metal bit as she nodded her head. Out in the air, high on this horse, for a while I was released from the earth and even when she was just walking quite slowly, I felt I might be flying. For a moment on my horse I could be like my sister and become something other, too. There was so much silence out there in the fields, apart from my big brave horse, that it was as if the air crackled around me, the trees and the hill beyond, the green cut out against the white sky like shapes the children might snip with their scissors. It was the middle of the day but it was by now mid-December and the light had that thin, diluted quality, as if darkness might overcome it at any moment, even though it should be light until at least four o'clock.

My horse dropped her head and snorted, reaching her muzzle down into the flood that covered the end of the field and I kicked her forward, as Galahad or Gawain might have done as they rode out on their quests into the forest where the frost was undisturbed. She walked bravely forward so that she was chest-deep in the dark black water.

I turned her around, walking her again and again through the deep water, concentrating on the sound of her hooves splashing and crashing and the feeling of how sure her feet were. She was brave. I thought of the descriptions I had read to the children the night before from the book about Arthur's knights who carried swords with highly polished hilts. Their horses were sometimes described as steeds and now I felt my horse might be such an animal too. A little stream called Rosie Brook runs alongside the field, meandering around blackthorn trees and willows that weep into the water over half-broken bridges with baler twine holding wicket gates together. I rode along the headland, the strip of land between the brook and the edge of the cold hard ploughed field, and suddenly in front of me a sharp dart of brown fur revealed two deer, not so big, moving fast and then stopping as they turned stock-still to face me. My horse stopped, mid splash, the dark water of this biggest puddle rippling around her hooves, and snorted, sending plumes of breath into the cold winter air. Then the deer darted forward again over the crest of a small hill, and I felt the lightest I had in several days as wonder came over me, for maybe that was her, who I was looking for all, all, all, all, all, all, all, all, all, all the time. There was no wind and the trees stripped of their leaves were still and the long rough grass growing on the headland was still and apart from the brown of the deer vanishing the world looked black around me.

'Be with me. Show me you are with me, show me you haven't gone,' I was shocked to hear my voice saying, that deeper voice which had stopped sounding completely like my own although I was not sure how my sister could have found her way into my voice box. All around there was silence and stillness until suddenly my horse snorted again and jumped forward, a gust of cold, ferocious wind in the still air spooking this animal and I thought: Was that a message?

But even if that gust of wind had been her – if my sister truly had transformed herself in death into the elements of the world around me – my mind absolutely could not contort into the right position to imagine that she actually was an element. Her body was still in the refrigerator in Stroud and I could not think where her soul was. If I looked up to the sky where night looked as if it might fall at any moment, even in the middle of the day, I imagined the whole sky was taken up with her face. I wondered if she was looking for me too. I wondered if she was missing me as I missed her. Was she looking for me? Did she miss me too? And when I thought of her face I was even more confused. Was she laughing and smiling at me or was she crying as I was? I wanted to see her laughing, or at least smiling since laughing might be a bit too rough for me right now, but I didn't think that could be possible yet. And I also absolutely did not want to see her crying. I did not want to imagine she had any pain. I didn't want to see her suffering although I couldn't imagine how she could not be, so great was the loss all around. I would have been confused too, I think, to see her blank face, so although with every part of me I wanted her face in the sky, I didn't know how it could be there. This further confusion about where my sister was made me feel scared and stupid that I had ever imagined myself as Galahad and that made me start crying again as I rode onwards.

When I turned my horse around the edge of the field to walk back along Rosie Brook, I felt absolutely terrified.

I couldn't stop crying and I didn't want to either. I wanted to scream like someone being murdered, because that was the kind of pain I felt: as if my own soul had been ripped from my body too. In the brook the brown water was swirling and when I looked down there I did not see the twigs and old leaves caught in the edge of the brambles but instead I saw her face and her hands with her palms upwards as if she was pressing from inside the water trying to get out. She looked urgent and not happy or peaceful and she was looking past me, trying to get out of the water, which seemed to me to be holding her under. I didn't like seeing her, my sister, trapped there under the surface of the cold water, so I kicked my horse forward to try to get back home to the light and colour, because I was scared and alone and death was surrounding me.

My horse stepped sideways around a pile of burnt sticks where there had been a bonfire in a far corner of the field, but the blackened ends of the wood left there, all charcoaled, scared me too because they looked like my sister's bones, and the blackened felled stump of a tree I rode past might have been her too. I wanted to get back home away from this but there was black plastic wrapped around an abandoned hay bale and I thought it was her body, wrapped and left out in the field. And I screamed, again, up on my horse, because I was very frightened, scared and alone, but more than anything because I wanted to go back in time, to the moment before death when she was alive, and to be in that world with her in it, not this new one without her.

I didn't talk to Pete or the children when I got back home, ripping my wet clothes off and folding myself into bed, enclosing myself into the darkness as my body shook and I cried again. It was 2 p.m. and I slept for two hours, dreaming that my hands had become all puffed up like hers did as I held them in the last hour of her life. I dreamed I was dying like my sister had died and when I woke I was still trapped in a dream in which I was floating face down in a deep puddle of sewage.

I did not know where my fear would take me and I was very afraid. I wanted to be told by someone how to live and what to think and how to walk through each day. Someone must have an answer to this intolerable feeling of deep heart pain. I couldn't find a guide anywhere so I started sending myself text messages as clues.

If you keep talking to her perhaps she won't let go.

If you talk to her she might hear. Talk to her. She won't let go.

As well as the conversations and messages, there were other words to deal with in those days after death. Some of these were formal terms like those on the certificates and forms that must be completed or collected to prove that the death has happened. Six days after she had died, I stood alone in my room holding her death certificate. Those words were mostly black and white. They were stiff and printed out in Times New Roman and they seemed to forbid me to move towards the new world that they described.

Name **Eleanor Rose GIFFORD.**
Maiden surname of woman who has married **STROUD.**
Date and place of death **Eighth December 2019, Gloucestershire Royal Hospital, Gloucester.**
Occupation **Circus Proprietor.**
Cause of death **Metastatic breast cancer.**

And at the end, this piece of paper carefully told me:

> WARNING: CERTIFICATE IS NOT EVIDENCE
> OF IDENTITY.

I held the certificate in my hands and I read it and reread it as though I was looking for truth in it because the only thing that was becoming clear to me now was that I was searching for something. Something incalculably precious had been lost. Something glimmering and golden and white and beautiful was gone. I didn't even know what the shape of this thing was or what it was, but I could feel its absence all around me, every moment I was awake, and a definite heaviness in my sleep too. I also knew I was very afraid of where the search would take me and so the CERTIFICATE might be a clue.

I ran my hand over the paper, which still felt warm from printing. Formal letterings and straight lines marked out boxes where the words had to go. The words of death were typed into these boxes, which was a good thing. The boxes were helpful to anyone who has just been with their dead relative, since after this kind of pain, people's handwriting can be too wobbly for them to be expected to fill the form out themselves with a biro, as if it's just a regular form at the dentist. My father once showed me a picture of the signature of Guido Fawkes just before he was taken to be tortured for his part in trying to blow up the Houses of Parliament. It looks like this:

The second signature was three days later, after he had been tortured in the Tower, and it looks like this:

Pain had broken his writing in half so that there was nothing of him left. Guido Fawkes had almost vanished. Looking at my sister's death certificate I thought about this and realized that was maybe why it had such clear boxes: to contain the pain. I had tried to write a note to Evangeline's teacher two days after my sister died and I could not do it because the pain in my body made my writing illegible, as if I had been on the rack too.

I could not find anything I was looking for in the certificate because when I looked at the typed words, they seemed to float away from me and into the room, vanishing. I thought the certificate itself might be wrong, and indeed that warning was written into it: 'CERTIFICATE IS NOT EVIDENCE OF IDENTITY.' Yes, the certificate must be wrong. She was not dead. My sister was not the deceased and the very certificate I was holding was telling me that. If I stopped concentrating so hard on this piece of paper in my hand with all its typed black words I could go backwards to the days before 8 December 2019 and I could live again in the past where my sister still existed. And in that moment, I realized that was what I was looking for: a way of returning into my life as it had been and as it had felt when she was alive in it.

I put the death certificate away in the back of a cupboard in my bedroom, under a deep pile of envelopes and postcards so that I would not have to see it again. Then I left my room to go back downstairs to the children. I was feeling more certain, since the certificate had told me, that the truth of her death might not actually be real. I wanted to feel certain and not like Guido, but when I moved along the upstairs corridor I gasped like someone had run a blade into my veins, because the sudden memory of unbearable loss that struck me was a physical sensation so acute it could not be pretended away. Sound and motion around me were horribly distorted; the scrape of a kitchen chair from the wooden floor downstairs shocked me as if it was happening right in my ear, but when my daughter Dolly appeared at her bedroom door I felt as if the edges of her were blurring and her words were in the wrong order: 'OK Mum you are?'

My feet flapped like deflating balloons as I walked down the stairs. With each step I felt as if new scaffolding was collapsing inside me. Everything had been ransacked. The certificate had ransacked me and every moment was hurting.

In the kitchen there was a bunch of white roses and a tray of macaroni cheese a friend had left, and beside that a toppling pile of letters. They had started arriving straight after my sister's death: an avalanche of sorrow and sadness. I walked around the kitchen, ripping each envelope open, reading the words as I poured milk into coffee and picked up plates covered in crumbs from the table. I did not want to sit at the table or on a sofa in a quiet room and read them. If I did that, and gave them my space and time, I was very scared they would take on the formality or even the power of the death certificate I had been trying to deny, and that might make them come true. The sadness in them might overwhelm everything and, since it took all my concentration at that moment to walk upstairs and down again, I couldn't be having that. Because although I had hidden the death certificate, I could feel it, black and burning in the cupboard in our bedroom, above the kitchen.

So I only skimmed through a lot of the letters because reading the words hurt too much.

Her death

I cannot begin to imagine your pain

Such shock and sadness

So much sorrow

Her bravery

So sorry for your loss

Her death

I cannot imagine your loss

So sorry for this suffering

Her death comes as a terrible shock

Terrible sorrow and grief

Her death

Such dark days for you

Her loss is beyond belief

Her death

Unimaginable loss and darkness

The sadness you must be feeling

Deep regret and loss

Her death

So brave

Cannot begin to imagine how you are feeling

The words stepped out towards me but I kept moving around the kitchen, because I reckoned that if I kept moving, and perhaps did not finish all the letters, just glanced at them instead, then they might fail to imprint themselves on to my life too, in the same way that I'd tried to trick the death certificate by hiding it in a place I never normally looked. Because my sister, golden and glowing just six days before, couldn't be dead. She was somewhere, I thought, as I dropped letters full of words I did not want to read around me, leaving the envelopes on the floor.

Some of the letters told me they were so sorry I had lost her, and I could feel this opening something in my heart that made it beat faster. Surely if something is lost, it can be found again, if you search hard enough? Pray to St Anthony, our mum would say to us when we lost precious things when we were little children together. This was before we were teenagers, before her accident, before she stopped being able to talk or walk or communicate in any way or look after herself or us at all and when she still knew who she was and who we were.

If my sister was lost, then surely St Anthony would return her to me? Mum always said to save the prayers to him for something very special. So, for example, do not squander prayers to St Anthony to get him to try to find your lost felt-tip pen lids, but he might help if you prayed to him after losing a very precious and old toy given to you by someone you loved very much.

Other letters referred to my sister as having passed away, which also dug a small fishing hook into my brain that I didn't like. 'Passed around' might have been more fitting, with its spirit of generosity and hospitality, conviviality even. Because although I had lost her, she also seemed to be everywhere suddenly, in these letters and text messages and WhatsApps and Instagram posts and messages which all expressed an unbounded love, respect, awe for my sister. She was clearly, obviously, being thought about in many people's hearts and heads. A sense of her must be in all those people's homes and deep in the conversations they were having with one another. She must have been very present to those people.

'Lost' holds hopelessness alongside hope. I had lost a gold bracelet Pete had given me when I was forty but found it in a drawer a year later. Something lost would be found.

'I lost my young daughter earlier this year,' one letter said to me, but I did not read any further, folding the letter quickly, like an official document, sliding it back into the envelope, then shuffling all the letters back together like a gigantic pack of cards which I might be about to deal to see if I could change fate. I kept thinking of the woman with the lost little child and, in my confusion, as I walked through the rest of that day as if entirely absent, I felt we might be able to join forces in the hunt. She must be here somewhere, my sister! She was a precious important person, worthy of all St Anthony's prayers, so if I looked hard enough I would find her. And your little daughter, precious pearl, can't have gone far either; she's just lost but might be found.

At lunchtime and for much of the rest of that afternoon, I was not really there. I ate baked potatoes and roast chicken with Pete and the children, but in my head I was ransacking the house, looking for the lost loved one. As I sat at the

kitchen table and passed the butter and salt and helped
Lester cut his potato skin, I could feel myself running
through the house, calling my sister's name as I do when
I've lost one of the children. I'm laughing at first, searching
under beds, behind closed cupboard doors, and again and
again I am calling out her name with a certainty I will find
her as I whoosh a duvet back, thinking she must be there,
she must be here somewhere, so I call her name, call her
name, call her name. *Come back! Where are you? Don't
let me lose you, my sister, where are you? Where are you?*
And then I start to realize I cannot find her anywhere, and
so my voice becomes hysterical, screaming. My brain
would not compute this feeling that I would never find her
again, so I told myself quiet things no one else could hear
to reassure and calm it and I continued eating roast chicken.

The timing of when things happened in those first seven
days after I had been in the room with my sister and death
was important. Like the days after birth, when the newborn
arrives in life but is not yet a day old, then one, then three,
then five, then a week, I was counting my sister's days since
death and also the quantity of days since I had been in
close proximity to death. After I gave birth to all my children I'd had this sense of disorientation and dislocation. It
might be possible to put this down to exhaustion, but I
believe it also comes from getting very close to the brink
between life and death. After my children arrived I cried a
lot too, and maybe that was because of my proximity to
birth, which, like death, is a deeply disturbing experience.

The two things are quite similar. And in the same way that after my children's births I thought a lot about the edges of that experience and the place on the brink I'd stepped into when they were being born, now I thought about death a lot of the time.

Being present at birth is disturbing and should be disturbing because of the extremities of it, and I was seeing that it was the same with death. I saw a separation between the absence of my sister and the fact that we had been in the room with death. Death had found its way around us, settling as imperceptible but present as dark dust, coating everything, even the inside of my heart and the crevices of my soul, the furthest corners of which I'd never felt before, even after my mother had died. I had felt something profound then but different, since she had been ill and unable to speak or communicate for twenty-two years before she died. She was also much older than my sister, at the end of her life, unlike my sister who might have been in the middle of hers had death not arrived. And my sister had been so very alive so very recently. We had not seen death coming for her. Not at all. And when I tried to get a brush out and sweep the dust away, sweep the darkness away, I realized it was impossible. The dust smudged over all the surfaces around me and even if I'd rubbed at it with a damp cloth it wouldn't have come off. It had marked everything, making things that were shiny and coloured or golden now dull and tarnished. I felt trapped in a dark cage in a dark room which enclosed me all the time, wherever I was, even if I was standing in the middle of my kitchen in front of the turquoise cooker as the children unpacked tinsel from a cardboard box and wrapped it all around the table and around the coloured kitchen chairs and then all around themselves, laughing. Even as they did this, lit by their own dazzle, I was inside a black cage, watching them from a distance.

This feeling of death around me all the time was separate from my grief. Grief was an emotion that I had to live through. It became a very active verb, although what it often made me want to do was lie down on the floor. Sometimes I cried so much I thought I'd be sick, and at other times I had to brace myself with my head in my hands, as I had when I had given birth to my children, when the pain suddenly hit me. Grief was happening to me all the time. Quite often I shivered and shook as if I had a plague, even in front of the wood burner in the pink playroom at home, and tears ran down my face and choked me; sometimes snot from my nose mixed with the salt water on my face. I looked strange. I behaved in a strange way. I sounded strange. I was strange. I was often not like a mother. I tried to explain this to Evangeline, when she came running to me and I was all empty and hurting, not welcoming and nurturing, ready to soothe and console her as I hope I usually am as her mum.

'It's OK, Evangeline,' I told her as she sat on my lap when I was crying. 'I just miss her, and I am grieving.'

But if grief was a very active word, death was something else. A noun, or even a proper noun, I was thinking of like this:

I am acquainted with Death.

Rather than this:

I am acquainted with death.

I had seen and faced the biggest proper noun in my life at that time, Death, and I could not simply forget it and move quietly on. If you met someone really important, someone who you knew at that moment was the love of your life, or your newborn child, or even a major and important and famous person – Michelle Obama, for example – the chances are they would make such a huge impression on you that you would mentally mark the day you met him/her. You might say to your friend afterwards: 'Wow, that really changed my life, when I met [insert significant name] last week.'

That was how I felt now. There was the loss of my sister, but there was also the meeting with Death. It had worked its way into me, like grit in an oyster, small and imperceptible but now an absolute part of me I couldn't rid myself of.

So when I got to seven days after my sister had gone, I felt a huge compulsion to do something to honour her and to recognize that moment. Pete had had to go to America for work. Some of my friends were worried about this, and were almost shocked, but it wasn't as if Death was suddenly going to pay the mortgage and fill the fridge and insure the car. He had to go. And I was OK with that. Pete is part of me like my sister is part of me. Even when we're apart, or even when we are in the middle of a massive argument, we're still completely together, even physically. Also, going about the active process of grieving is very time-consuming and requires a lot of concentration. To a certain extent, I wanted to be on my own.

So, I was on my own with the children, Pete was on his way to New York but it was Sunday and it was 3.47 p.m. and we were moments away from seven days, a week, having passed since my sister had died. I knew it was acutely important to be doing something at that moment – 4.20 p.m. – to honour what had happened and not, for example, to be emptying the bins or looking for a lost shoe. I drove with my younger children, Dash, Evangeline and Lester, as my elder children Jimmy and Dolly were with their dad, to White Horse Hill, a big boulder of a hill about two miles away that rises within sight of our house so that I face it every time I open the front door. It was so cold, and we parked near the top of the hill at 4.09 p.m., and when I opened the car doors, the children were screaming and crying as I had been for many of the days before then. I took Dash and Lester by the wrists and pulled them, resisting hard, up the incline, to the Neolithic fort on top of the hill as they bawled at me. Evangeline ran ahead of me, her yellow hair whipping around her small face as we arrived at the top at 4.16 p.m.

'We are doing this to honour her,' I said to them very loudly to drown out their screams.

Sharp points of black crow sliced through the belly of milky grey sky around us and at 4.19 p.m. at the top of the hill, I let go of Dash and Lester's wrists. There was no one else there, apart from a distant walker on the far side of the incline in purple nylon walking gear. Then I opened my arms and it was 4.20 p.m. and I stood in the wind as Dash ran away from me, and Lester lifted his head to watch me, and I shouted her name into the wind and the air. Time moved forward and I could feel it around me, as the hour of her death rushed further backwards into the past to where I really wanted to be. Evangeline watched me too and I know I was scaring her. I didn't want to scare her. I didn't want to feel this undone but since it was all I felt, I knew I needed to be this way too.

Later, when we were home, there was a letter, handwritten, posted through the door. The person who had written the letter had left an email address and a phone number in case 'you wanted to talk at any point' or there 'was anything I can do to help'. The letter was so kind but also scared me a little as I imagined it demanded something of me – a return email, for example, explaining what could be done to help. If someone could have shown me a way back through the portal in time, so that I could get back to before, when my sister was alive, that would definitely have helped. But I couldn't really think of anything else there could be to do.

When I looked up from the letters, Lester was standing in the kitchen, wearing one shoe.

'Trouble is sitting in a bubble,' he said quietly.

Eight days after we had left the hospital, I went to London to see my father and my stepmother and think about my sister's funeral. When I texted my father with this word 'funeral' it felt all wrong. I wanted to write 'the event' or 'on the day' or something more opaque. We were all looking at the same day in the future and so to actually identify 'the funeral' wasn't completely necessary.

In my most recent adult existence I like to believe that I have pretty much pushed my life in a direction I have chosen it to go. My teenage life ruptured when I was sixteen and I found myself then for a long time in rooms I did not want to be in, but recently I've been more or less where I want. The sudden arrival of these new words in my life reminded me of the days when I had no agency at all. Death swooping in had taken all of us into a place we didn't want to go. Those very, very painful words like 'coffin', 'hearse', 'crematorium or burial?', 'eulogy', 'wake' were suddenly part of many of the messages we had to send one another in the days after death: a new language and vocabulary which I didn't want to use. If I was talking to Pete, sometimes I'd rush through a word like 'hearse' so that I didn't have to really think about it, but at other times I forced myself to say the words very slowly: 'Crem-at-or-i-um'. 'Coff-in'. 'Bur-i-al'.

There. You see? You can say them. They are powerful but they are also simply words. Be brave.

However, contained in those words were decisions we had to make, which was why I went to my father's house to talk with him and my stepmother. My father is a brave person and he always encouraged my sister and me to examine our lives, read stuff that would help us understand other people's lives and also to write or create things that would help us communicate what life felt like. Our mother did this too, although the way she taught us was probably more physical than my father. My dad encouraged us to read a lot and my mother taught us about physical bravery, which (I later understood) can translate into emotional bravery. But they made us search for things, and then when what happened to our mother became part of our everyday lives – her accident and brain damage – it also meant we were always, always looking for something quite serious in life. For example, about seven years ago, my sister and I went to a showground for an event called Your Horse. It was supposed to be a big event with horse displays and people doing dressage clinics and show-jumping lessons in front of big crowds in big arenas. The whole event had sounded interesting on the marketing material, but when we got there we hardly saw any real horse clinics. Instead, it felt more like big barns full of stalls and stalls and stalls with people selling horse equipment that was mostly very sparkly and pink. There were pink bridles and head collars and brushes, hoof picks, riding boots all covered in pink plastic or pink coatings or pink glitter. It wasn't what we had been looking for at all, and we walked between the stalls and all the pinkness and we both knew we were look-ing for something which was more meaningful and important. Right in a distant corner we found a small stall selling old prints of horses and second-hand books called things like *Teaching Your Carriage Horse*, *My First Pony* and *World of Horses*. We'd had quite a few of those books when we were children. Right amongst them we found a book about Gypsies and what had happened to them during the

Holocaust. After we'd found this book, we both felt relieved. It hadn't been a waste of time after all. Amid all the pink plastic we had found some kind of vitally important truth about human experience.

I thought about this as I crossed London. A lot of the time, even when I was talking about something else, like which train I should catch or who might pick the children up from school, the thing that my brain really was saying to me was whereareyou whereareyou whereareyou whereareyou whereareyou whereareyou whereareyou, like an extremely loud and shocking alarm going off. Actually the sound in my head felt more like this:

WHEREAREY OUWHEREAR EYOUWHERE AREYOUWHE REAREYOUW HEREAREYO UWHEREAR EYOUWHERE

AREYOUWHE REAREYOUW HEREAREYO UWHEREARE YOUWHERE AREYOUWH EREAREYOU

I think I was doing quite well as it's not easy going about any kind of normal business in a normal way with that kind of alarm unstoppable in your head; it's certainly not easy to do things like buy train tickets. However, despite this, I think I looked relatively normal. I wore white trainers and black jeans and a black coat, as there was clarity in dressing in black, it required no decisions of me, but my face was red and puffy because being so close to death meant that I still cried a lot of the day.

'**LONDON LOVES LIFE!**' a red and white sign exclaimed, reflected backwards in the shine of the train window on the underground as I tried to concentrate on my white trainers to make the whereareyou alarm stop. London loves life, I repeated to myself, but what I wanted to know was what did London think of death?* How could London be going about its loving, exciting life with traffic lights changing and waiters clearing cafe tables and electric doors in shops opening and closing and opening again while heat blew out from their interiors, while death was working its way through my life? How could London go on loving life if my sister was dead?

'Loving life is impossible,' I said aloud as I walked down the streets to my father's home, but by the time I arrived there I felt quite cheerful, since the walking was good and it had put a silencer on the alarm in my head. The walk had also made me think of Galahad again and how much I would have liked to have him riding along beside me. What a sight that would have been: a knight on a horse riding down the King's Road (the right name for it, in that case). The sound of his horse's hooves on the pavement would have made me happy and it occurred to me that making a knight on a horse ride through a city was exactly the kind of thing my sister organized, very regularly, in her circus life.

When I got to their house, waving farewell in my head to Galahad, who rode on down the Embankment past the buses, I wanted to clasp and carefully hug and treasure my stepmother and father as if they were glass icons, because I was so relieved to see them and find them alive. For a while I had been thinking that death might have taken everything. Instead I felt light and excited, my palms sweating as we

---

* In December 2019, before the virus, the old life was still normal.

talked and they made me a cup of tea and we stepped around the fact, carefully, that we were here to plan my sister's fun-er-al.

Oh dear.

There: the word felled me again. I was with my father, laughing, and then suddenly, death was on my back, this time like a big cat, its claws and jaws in me as I grimaced and shook with pain, trying to get the violence of it away from me, please, make the pain stop, where are the knights with their fearsome flashing swords to help me now? Galahad, come back.

And maybe he heard me, because suddenly the pain passed as though someone strong had wrenched the massive dangerous animal off my back, and when I said thank you to my stepmother for the cup of tea she made, I heard that my voice was normal. I felt safe and relieved to be beside her, seeing her bare feet on the wooden boards of their warm home and her black shirt and beautiful black eyes.

After that we spent six hours going through the process of planning my sister's funeral. My father had already worked through much of it. He had thought of many poems and hymns my sister, his daughter, would have wanted. The only thing that I could really think of was that we should have T. S. Eliot and I asked for the hymn that had hobgoblins in it and the one that sounded like 'By the Rivers of Babylon' by Boney M. The one I meant was 'On Jordan's Bank the Baptists Cry' but I could not remember the name of it and anyway, as things turned out, we were not allowed it as it was one for Advent. My sister's funeral was to be at Gloucester Cathedral in January, after Advent, and we could not make up the rules. As we sat and talked about it, I realized that the funeral would be the last real gift we gave my sister, and so I told my father I wanted to give a eulogy. And I wanted to be one of six people who would carry her coffin too. I felt as if the height of my pain would also be a measure (to me at least, understand this was a completely personal challenge) of the height of how I missed her, and bearing the weight of her body felt like a way of truly feeling this.

Later, from the train on the way home, I had to speak to the undertaker. He told me he had some things I needed to consider.

'You need to think about her dress to be buried in.' And: 'You should consider if there is anything you would like to add to your sister's coffin.'

Yes, I told him, there is. Letters and drawings and some small things that had been important to her that I wanted to go on with her.

He told me that letters could be dropped off at the funeral home as late as the night before the funeral.

'Before the coffin is sealed,' he said to me.

Afterwards, I stared at my phone screen all the way home until the train reached Didcot. These were the things I would think about over Christmas, which was now a few days away.

Can we do a lot of lying around in blankets drinking fine wine?

was a WhatsApp message my now dead sister had sent the group ★Christmas in Wales★ which my sisters and I and our children had started in October, two months and one day before she died. Hers had been the first message in the group: Excited!! 🎈🎈🎈. She had also written, We can make stuff from the hedges for decorations. I'll order a turkey today.

Now, instead of planning Christmas in Wales, I was writing a letter to send her *before the coffin is sealed.*

Chapter 2

I Have to Look Away and I Don't Want to Walk into the Forest

I went into the kitchen early in the morning. In the silence of the room I felt calmer and safer. Big bright noises around me were still extremely disorientating at this point, three-quarters of the way through December, but in the kitchen there was peace to be found. There were the hyacinth bulbs in pots that forced their way through the darkness of the soil and made a sudden explosion of pink and blue. They smelt so strong, almost synthetic, but they filled the air and there was a consolation for me in simply being there, alone, not expected to say or do anything, not expected to be anything to anyone else.

One morning, after the children had broken up for Christmas but before they were out of bed, I quickly pulled on my clothes and walked out into the fields beside our house. The willow tree there was stripped bare of its leaves shaped like little fishes and the moon was still in the sky, though not so big and white as it had been, and the air smelt cold, of first frost melting. There was a little crunch of the thinnest ice on a puddle, and I heard crows making their hard cawing sound but I could not see them as I walked through frost-stiff grass, unsure of where I was going or even whether I needed to know where I was going. It didn't matter. There was nowhere to go that mattered now.

I climbed the cold metal gate near the churchyard and walked down the edge of the headland running around the field, where there is no footpath. For a few moments, a black cat I see in the village followed me, but then vanished when I turned around to look for it. Instead, on the horizon closest to me I could see the stiff outline of an oak tree that stands in the middle of the field but I didn't walk across to it, since the land is ploughed, but instead walked on down the edge of the field, skirting the metal fence which divides the land from a deep cutting, where a train track runs close to our house. My breath was warm in the air and although my hands were cold I didn't put them into my pockets as I wanted to feel exposed to the elements. I imagined this might give me a clearer sense of what I was feeling and how to withstand what was happening. Then I became aware of the barn owl I often see, dipping and swooping in that low-flying way, just ahead of me along the hedge. I stopped, holding my breath for a moment, willing the bird towards me, and it worked, because when I stood as still as

I could the bird passed, and I caught a glimpse of its big, empty eyes looking out into the darkness, almost close enough to feel the beat of its white wings. Seeing the round, startling flash of the face of the bird so close up brought to mind a man I had seen flat out on the concrete beside a dual carriageway. I had glimpsed him in the same way: very quickly, since I was driving, and there were two cars that had stopped beside him with their lights on. On the edge of the carriageway there was some twisted metal that moments before had been his bicycle, but it was the man's face and the shape of his body that stayed with me, even from that single moment as I passed him, pressed against the concrete, his arms and legs outstretched and his body like a star. I saw him ten years before I had watched my sister die but I had thought about him often, that dead man, in the years afterwards. It had shocked me to think that I didn't know him and yet I was one of the first people to see him dead. Afterwards I tried to look him up. I wondered if he had had a family who was waiting for him and for a while I wondered if I should try to contact them, but then I realized I had no idea what I would say to them, except that there seemed to be something important in having seen a man whose soul had been in his body just moments before. What I remembered was that he had looked peaceful, his face sideways to the concrete as if he was just resting there for a moment, and I had wanted his family or anyone who had cared about him to know this. The calm, wide-open way that the owl looked towards me reminded me of him for a moment before it swooped off and was gone.

As I turned the corner at the end of the field, returning to the house where the children would be waking and the noise of the day would begin, I thought about what lay ahead. I realized that other people might instruct me but I walked alone. And I was scared by this, just as I had felt extremely scared by my feelings in the landscape as I rode my horse in those days soon after my sister's death. The ground beneath my feet felt unsteady and death was disorientating me. There was no map I could follow. I felt a quickening in my heart, my pulse was racing and I knew this was because of the enormity of the task I faced.

As I turned to the house, six crows alighted from the oak tree. They were making that hard, cawing noise I had heard earlier and I knew that six crows together signified death. I paused for a moment, resting my hands on the cold metal of the gate. I realized I would be finding my way through a world in which the unimaginable must be imagined every day. Who was the brave one now?

After the dazzlingly painful colours of the first two weeks after my sister's death, and the oddness of Christmas, there was her funeral.

I have struggled to type the word so I have put it into a finer type for you now to make it less impactful. I had to close my eyes for a moment after I had typed it and look away.

I don't know how to write about it. I don't know how to tell you. It was beautiful but how do I describe something that was so beautiful and so terrible at the same time? I was there, in the cathedral, and I was also not there. And in the days afterwards, quite often I just lay on my bed, listening to my breathing, while feeling as cold and translucent as an iceberg, floating alone through a silent dark sea. Something like a huge bit of ice had sheared off from the edge of me; part of me was dissolving and becoming lost in the breathing sea, white ice inside me constantly melting, melting, melting. I was changing shape and could no longer feel the edges of myself. I didn't know what my intent or purpose was. The magnitude of having carried her coffin at my sister's funeral – my sister's funeral – moved through me like the deep, distant sound of ice cracking with nothing to witness it but the waves beneath.

Not absolutely all parts of me were cold and melting. Incredible sensations of colour appear in my mind when I remember her funeral. Her coffin, painted in burgundy, green, cream and with magic wrapped around it as it sat – as she lay – on a bank of flowers in the cathedral. The bright blue and shiny gold pattern of the new dress I had bought specially to match the blue and shiny gold dress covered in stars that she was wearing inside the coloured coffin, and the yellow of a burning candle I concentrated on as I spoke the words I wanted to say about my sister to that cathedral of people. After I finished the eulogy I sat back down and I stared at the pattern on my dress very hard, trying to make myself feel stable as I listened to my father talking with such grace and beauty and **bravery** about his dead daughter in his eulogy. The bright red of my cousin's red suede gloves as she held me around my shoulders. The clean brightness of the horses who pulled the hearse, their gleaming

whiteness and the bouncing golden-white plumes of feathers on their bridles, and the strange black feeling of the
storm that whipped up in a frenzy around the cathedral as
she was taken away. The hot flaming orange of the flares
beside the grave, which flickered so hard but did not blow
out, despite the storm and the rain, and the blackness of the
night as my sister's coffin was lowered into the ground, and
the bright white of the straps that took her down there. The
scarlet of the inside of someone's mouth when they were
talking to me, later, and the golden bubbles of their champagne, because there was a party, although I cannot
remember who that person was or who anyone was and I
cannot remember the party, apart from many many faces
close to mine. And a man with shoulder-length frizzy black
hair who wanted to touch me. He had an American accent
and I didn't know who he was.

'You look just like her. My God, you look the same as
your sister,' he kept repeating as he reached out to touch
my hair, then suddenly retracted his hand like I had
scorched his fingertips or I was a ghost he had touched.
Then he said, 'But you are much shorter than her.' He is the
only person I can clearly remember talking to.

Waking up the day after my sister's funeral was the bleakest
day of my life. I don't want to let you down but I will not
preserve it in beautiful words, and the weeks afterwards, the
bit that followed, made me feel cold and translucent. It was
mid-January by then and the ploughed field outside my bedroom was as hard as iron. The black lines of the oak tree in

the distant middle of the field scraped at the grey sky. There were always the blackest crows on the field, but sometimes Evangeline would come into the room, the bright aliveness of her skin and her hair all shimmering as she pressed her face against the windows. She liked to feel the glass on her face and look out to the field and search for foxes. There were lots of them in the field. They came up from a den in the railway cutting, pushing through the thick black brambles, hunting over the soil, noses down, twitching, their tails trailing, as if they knew everything they were doing and were confident of their place in that field, easy as anything. Evangeline's voice made a high, gasping sound when she saw them. Often she would spot one and then another and another. I didn't like looking at them so much. They had human faces and it was like they were staring right at me.

After the funeral it felt as if there was nothing valiant or brave left for me to do and instead I found myself worrying incessantly about all the people I really loved, afraid they might all die suddenly too. I felt overwhelmingly anxious that death might come for them as suddenly as it had for my sister, and I found myself speaking to my father and my stepmother every day. I wanted to talk to them because they are my friends but also I wanted to hear the sound of their voices to make sure they were not dead.

And I thought about sex a lot, because it stopped me thinking about death. Sometimes I wondered if, in between brief moments of doing small amounts of work or making packed lunches for children or feeding cats, we are all thinking about either death or sex all the time.

And sex was also a place in my head I could go to where the dark glitter of death had not settled. It was a whole new house full of rooms I could inhabit by pressing my naked body against Pete's. It was a way of asserting myself against death and the things it had done and what it had taken. When I could hear Pete's voice right inside my ear it was like being dropped into a moment within a different dimension where nothing had been lost, because nothing but that moment had ever existed. The renewal of being loved by Pete and the closeness I felt to him, whatever the circumstances, was like shiny silver coins suddenly pressed into my hands, little flashes of bright and valuable treasure I could secretly hold on to to survive, although it wasn't big enough to live on alone. To feel deeply loved by Pete could only make me think of life, and at those times death was nowhere, absolutely nowhere. And sex itself was a white place in my mind, still empty – although after the first time I had sex after my sister died, I felt so guilty. I had to press my face into the pillow so that Pete would not hear me crying.

One afternoon I was sitting on the edge of my bed staring into nothing and wondering if I still knew how to breathe when I realized I was actually gazing at the stack of books beside my bed. Books and books formed piles on the floor, which sometimes got moved around the house, so that the stack was ever-changing as I half read one or discarded another and replaced it with other books from other rooms in the house. Amongst them I could see the black spine of a book which drew my eyes towards it because I could see written there the word **Metaphysical**. Just the sound alone of that word struck a small chord inside me, as if it might describe this thing I had no words for that was happening to me. Written in biro inside the book, in small writing, was my sister's name, and 'St Paul's December 1990'. I read some of the poems and the words were difficult to understand but that suited how I felt, since I had become difficult to understand, so I just continued reading the difficult, strange, metaphysical words. Then I picked up my phone and looked up what metaphysical really meant:

The word **metaphysical** is a combination of the prefix of 'meta' meaning 'after' with the word 'physical' and is a philosophical concept used in **literature** to describe the things that are **beyond the description of physical existence** and which cannot be explained by science.

There was some small comfort in knowing I was living through metaphysics, although being *meta* didn't often make navigating the *physical* bit of life that much easier. The meanings of these poems were hard to grasp but I found the words consoling, and while my brain did not understand, my eyes focused on the idea of *'one blood made of two'* and landed on *'go tell court huntsmen that the king will ride'*, even if I understood nothing else. After

I'd been reading the poems for a while I realized the light had changed in my bedroom so it was getting later and I could hear Pete in the kitchen downstairs where I knew the children would be yapping around him like hungry seals. I wanted to be with them and to be normal so as I walked downstairs I fixed my face into a less metaphysical shape and thought I would make a cup of tea and look fine, completely fine, and not mention death or my sister once, but just be my children's mother again. Our home needed a break from the petrol-blue wings of death that preoccupied me, always fluttering around me, in the side of my vision, if not actually obscuring everything around me.

It was warm in the kitchen; Pete had lit candles and drawn the long pink curtains and the brown wooden clock that had been my grandmother's was ticking so someone must have wound it up. A big pan of salty water with strands of spaghetti squirming around in it was boiling and bubbling on the cooker. Evangeline, Lester and Dash were bobbing around Pete, screaming with delight as he threw a strand of spaghetti on to the ceiling. When it stuck there, they laughed and jumped up and down with their hands over their mouths and I walked amongst them and tried to be less metaphysical, but a glass chip of memory in my brain moved with a scene in which my sister and I were children in the kitchen with my mum as she threw spaghetti on to the ceiling. I could feel the memory lodged there but I did not want to make it go deeper and become anything bigger. I knew that if I allowed that to happen the glass chip would cut me and start a bleed in my brain.

When Pete smiled at me, I thought that I smiled back looking quite normal, but when he really looked at my face I
saw his own fall.

'What's wrong?' he asked me, which gave me the same
feeling that I had when people said, 'How are you?'

I was trying so hard to be normal and not think about
memory or death but the feelings just overtook me, and
however hard I tried to stop it, a stupid grotesque sob came
out of my mouth because there was no way in the world I
could answer that question truthfully without really scaring
the children.

I thought about my relationship with my sister almost constantly. I didn't know how to imagine myself without her,
and when I did I heard a sound come from me, like a small
animal noise, registering loss and pain. When I talked
about her I was also trying out new ways to talk to her
which might help me reach back across death and communicate with her.

Where had all the time we had lived through together
gone? Something that really scared me and confused me was
my uncertainty about where I should save, and protect, even,
the precious times we had had together. No one else could
look after those memories. What would happen if I forgot
them or if there were big parts of them, of how moments *felt*,
that I could not remember without her to talk to? I wanted to
find a big silver chest with ruby-coloured stones studding it
where I could very, very safely store these things. If I forgot,
would that mean our childhood had never existed? Should I

make Pete sit down in the strange landscape I existed in and tell him absolutely everything I could remember which was inside me, so that the living person I trusted most with my life should know it all too? Would he be able to guard the feeling I had of my sister and me as little girls, sleeping in warm beds beside each other, learning to talk? Would he understand the feeling of being small children together and how much I had needed her to tell me when she shut her eyes at night in that shared room, so that I would not be in the darkness without her? Would he understand the feeling of walking through cold early-morning grass together barefoot, eating apples, when walking alone was something new? How could I properly convey the hot feeling of fighting each other, all the way through our lives, from when we were very small, which is still like thorns caught in my palms when I remember it? It's as much a part of me and her as everything else, all the love and all the words we spoke to each other through our forty-four and a half years together, and maybe the fights are part of the love, but how would I properly explain this to him when I didn't really understand it in words myself, only feelings?

The responsibility of being the sole keeper of these memories made me so afraid. What if I forgot? What if I failed?

There was a moment when my sister lay dying, when someone, a close family member, came to sit beside me. I had left my sister's bedside for a moment. There were a lot of people there in the final hours, who had arrived to see her alive one last time. A whole circus of people walked into her room, tears rolling and rolling. And so sometimes I left the room so that other people could sit with her for a moment, and I went to the family room, lined with plastic-backed chairs, and a view of Gloucester Cathedral rising above the city, which lay below it like screwed-up newspaper. I had been awake for thirty-three hours and the room was a little smudgy. This close family member sat beside me. She put her arm around me and hugged me.

'You will be all right. And it won't get any worse than this moment, now. This is the hardest moment.'

At that instant what she said had been very consoling, and her voice had been beautiful and she was beautiful, but now I thought about it, when I woke up, again, on another morning after her funeral, and I knew she had been completely wrong. I might have thought the days after her death were the worst ones, but the days after the funeral were much, much harder. In the days between her death and her funeral, I felt acutely connected to my sister. She was absolutely everywhere, in the flashing green eyes of a black cat and in the fast movement of a deer and in the rain that mixed with the water on my cheeks when I walked. Everywhere.

But now? Now that she was moving onwards, onwards, onwards, further away, what good could the days bring? A hurricane blew through my life and the door of normal life swung open, banging as it did so, but expecting me to walk through it.

Writing about these days is very difficult. For a few weeks in late January, this is what my life felt like:

Nothing.

Life had become nothing. Nothing was bright and I was like the stripped-bare, winter-naked trees. I couldn't see the shape of my life and didn't know how to fashion the shape of my family's lives as I once had. I was completely lost and inside me there was a void where once there had been my life. I'd given life my attention and heart and it had taken my sister and given me back death. I thought quite often about that reading which gets repeated at funerals or sent to you when someone you really love has died – the one that suggests death means that person has just slipped quietly away into another room. I was, I realized, rattling on the door of that room. I was leaning into it, slapping it with both my palms flat, imploring someone to open up and let me in too. I did not want to take my own life but I would like my own life to have been taken. I felt it would be exquisite to walk out of my house and not to come back. To vanish into the place I was before I was born and find my sister there.

I became so angry that the past was a place I could not go that instead I tried to imagine a place where I could give up all agency. I would not become a heroin addict or an alcoholic, but one night I sat in bed with my laptop and looked up how to join a cult. If I was part of a cult I could remain alive and yet give the direction of my life over to someone else. I didn't find anything useful and afterwards it occurred to me that this isn't the way to search for a cult to join since they're not going to advertise themselves on Gumtree or Instagram really, are they? Instead, perhaps I could take myself away to join a convent? There was something consoling in the idea of spending my days in the half-light, chanting prayers, hidden behind a habit and a veil, vanishing into a state of prayer, which might feel like a trance.

Instructions or information about how to exist with this new, unbearable loss did not seem to exist anywhere. I thought of images I had seen of satellites moving quietly far, far away in space and deep in time. I was floating some-where I didn't want to be. I was far from my sister and far from the life I knew.

One afternoon I was at home trying to stop my younger children throwing shoes at each other when one of my sis-ter's friends called me. I went into my room and shut the door. The woman wanted to know how I was and if I was, as she said, surviving. I wasn't dead yet. Her voice sounded bright. She said she had popped out of the office, and wasn't the sunshine lovely? In the background, I could hear the sound of a busy street. We talked about the funeral for a little bit. She said it was very beautiful and I said yes, yes it was. So many hundreds and hundreds of people.

Then she said: 'Be kind to yourself. Look after yourself. Your sister would want that. Remember all the joyful things you did together. You will find ways to live without her. Cook something she would have liked and enjoy that, or go for a walk in a place she loved. She would want you to do those things. And you are so strong. You have been through so much loss already. You will be even stronger and wiser. But be easy on yourself.'

Be easy on yourself. This might have sounded like some-thing straightforward but now felt like an imperative, a command to live well, and I didn't know how to do that. I felt so angry that my sister was gone. I did not want to be made to do the work to be stronger. I did not want to feel wiser or more resilient. I did not want to sanction what was happening by feeling that in some way I was learning from this loss. I wanted to fight against it. I had to resist telling this woman I would immediately swap everything I was learning about death, and life too, for her ignorance of it, if I could just get my sister back.

Outside my bedroom on the landing the children had finished throwing shoes and were now in their room having a spitting competition. I left them and walked through the house, trying to imagine enjoying places my sister and I had visited together. But I couldn't do it. The idea of wilfully taking myself to stand in certain places I remembered being with her when we were very happy – riverbanks, the high streets of small provincial towns, the Ridgeway, marshes, the city where we were born – felt like taking a small, very sharp, shiny, dangerous dagger and pushing it into the softest place in my throat, so I didn't do this. I thought of the woman telling me to cook something my sister would have liked, as if that could in some way be celebratory, but I could not even cook bacon in the black frying pan with chipped white enamel on the outside that had been our mum's without thinking of my sister, too, in her kitchen ('Bacon sandwich? Go on, Clo. Then we can go outside. You can borrow a coat, don't worry. Quick cup of tea?'), so I couldn't see how there was anything more elaborate she'd liked making – beef stew cooked with ginger or squash roasted with chilli or couscous with pomegranate seeds and orange zest covering it like jewels – that I could go anywhere near, let along *enjoy*.

After that, for a while I found that I was avoiding calls from people who wanted to know how I was. Instead I walked alone on the Ridgeway, which suited how I felt, which was grey and bleak and distant at this far point in the winter. Sometimes I saw muntjac deer, so small and lost as they shivered and crept across the huge landscape, but mostly I concentrated on the grey greasy chalk of the ancient track ahead of me. I know a tree in a forest makes a crashing sound when it falls because that was the sound I made as I walked alone and thought about my sister. There was an oak tree inside me and it crashed down as its roots were violently pulled up from the ground.

The hardness of late winter was relentless. It was the coldest and darkest part of the year. The field beyond the house was ploughed into brown clods and rooks sat on the fence, watching. The Christmas tree I had dumped in the garden on New Year's Day sat upside down in the blackened path of grass where Jimmy and his friends had had a bonfire, in a corner near the barn. It was half burnt, brittle branches like blackened bones resolutely surviving despite the teenage destruction wreaked upon it. On Facebook, people started posting that it was lighter in the evenings now, no longer dark at 5 p.m., they said. But the light was thin, it was constantly cold, and if not cold, then always wet, since it rained, incessantly, like vats and vats of tears pouring down across the world. Pete said this was definitely climate change and soon flooding would become normal around our home. It seemed only to stop raining for one day in

January, which was the day Pete and I and the children went back to my sister's grave for the first time. I hadn't been there since seeing her coffin lowered into the ground with the white straps and as we walked up the steep hill to the place where she was buried, I felt very afraid. There were flowers still there and cards with messages to her from many of her friends. There were some flowers in the shape of a cross with ivy woven through them and bunches of orange and white chrysanthemums. They had been there for almost three weeks and the petals were broken. I could not look at the flowers a friend had sent that spelt out the letters of her name. The flowers were so fucking poignant, I could not stand looking at them. Seeing her name on her grave like this felt beyond supernatural. I was staring directly at something I should never have seen and somehow I felt that if I looked at it too long I might be betraying my sister and somehow betraying life itself. Those things exposed life as a ruined, dark, frightening place.

I could not stay long at the grave. Instead, we walked back down the hill and sat outside the pub in the village to eat lunch, since it was suddenly a very sunny day. We sat in front of big white plates of roast beef, looking up to the hill where my sister's house was, on the opposite side of the valley, and I felt as sad and empty as it is possible for a person to feel.

Later that night I went to the children's bedroom to read to them. As they jumped from one bed to another I looked through their bookshelves, picking up a very faded old copy of *Fantastic Mr Fox*, with a picture of a cartoon fox on the front beside a big moon. The pages were old and slightly stuck together – successive cups of hot milk set beside children's beds had been slopped on them. The front cover fell open at a page with writing on it. There were our names together in biro: my name and my sister's name and then, in our mother's writing, 'Love from Mum and Rick Christmas 1977'. I made that noise again, that small, animal noise of loss, and I could actually feel the outer edges of my heart inside my chest constricting as the past fell away like a bundle over the side of a cliff, faster and faster, vanishing out of reach.

I closed the book, pushing my mum's writing back into the bookcase, and left the children jumping from one bed to another. I needed to sit quietly on my own and think about that petrol-blue beauty in the black wings of the crows I'd seen alighting in the field. At that point I was very afraid I'd fail in the task ahead, and fail as a mother, too.

Chapter 3

An Animal Caught in a Trap

One afternoon, before the children came back from school, I locked my bedroom door to study photographs of my sister. I needed to do it alone, when the children were out of the house, since I knew this was a precarious edge to wilfully take myself to. I knew it would hurt and I needed to feel that pain of looking directly at my sister without the children anywhere nearby needing me.

Many of the images existed within my phone so were always close to me, but I also had several big bags of prints that I had carried around with me since I was a teenager. I knelt on the floor with my computer open, flicking through image after image of the life I had lived around my sister. And I pulled the photographs out from the back of a cupboard, searching through hundreds of them, spreading them on the floor around me. I had some very old pictures of us as children together, in gardens or on beaches, sometimes looking serious, sometimes happy with wonky smiles and tufty hair, in faded shorts or patchwork dresses and knee-length socks and brown buckled sandals. I made myself look at these beside recent pictures of her on my computer, just the summer before – *a few months before* – outside a Spar shop in a village on holiday, all our children lined up beside us after we'd blown their minds buying them more than all the sweets they had asked for. My sister was wearing a long red skirt in the photograph, bright white trainers despite the fact we'd just walked across salt marshes to get to the shop, big shades, her hair cropped short and bleached blonde. Everyone was smiling or laughing, and there were more pictures from the same trip, on a bench outside a friend's house, my sister with a sketch pad in her hand as our children lay in a pile around her, laughing. There were many more I scrolled through, some that I had photographed from my father's albums, pictures he had taken when we were children and then young adolescents, wearing matching outfits at a party, and another walking together across a stubble field, one on a mountain in Italy, that last summer before Mum's accident. I had to put those photographs down because beyond that last summer I could feel a wall of loss and the bright colours of trauma lying like a lake before us. Very, very carefully I studied more pictures from just before my sister's diagnosis, in the summer of 2015, looking for clues while trying to remember what that moment felt like.

When I had been staring at the pictures for a while, I sat back on my heels, and exhaled, only realizing then that I had been holding my breath. I stood up, rubbing my forehead because my ears were ringing, leaning over to open the window so that I could get some more air, but that wasn't enough. I left the images spread over the floor and went downstairs, trying to make myself breathe deeply, trying to keep my fists from clenching.

I pulled on boots, climbing the fence beside our house, walking quickly down the hedgerow running to the church nearby, wet boots pushing through rain-soaked grass, sodden with deep winter. The ground gave beneath my feet because it was so wet but there was also a boring reassurance to it, unlike the light vertigo I'd felt looking back at the pictures of myself at sixteen. The person I saw from before Mum's accident, before that moment of intense, beyond-bearing loss, was a different person. I walked on, pushing my way along the hedgerow, trying to arrange my brain into a shape I could, if not understand, at least contemplate without having to look away.

Mum's accident proved to me that loss forges you in a crucible into someone different. The hot sparks of trauma mould you into a new shape: one that you resist even though it might be stronger and more able to withstand force applied to it than the previous version of you. Even now, in mid-life, I have some friends whose parents and siblings are all alive and undamaged by accidents or the vertigo of loss and sometimes I look at them and wonder: What does that feel like? To have that certainty right into mid-life, and even, in some people's cases, late mid-life, like those with very, very elderly parents and healthy siblings, for whom death and loss are not absolutely everywhere all the time, hovering and ready to take absolutely everything from you. I wondered if I felt more dead or more alive than those people, only I didn't have time to decide.

As I reached the end of the field, beyond the church where the field falls away and our house is no longer in sight, I saw something bright and vivid, matted brown fur tugging back in the grass. Slowly I knelt down to where a rabbit with black, bulging shiny eyes quivered and shook, wrenching backwards, caught in a strand of bright silver wire from a broken fence. When the rabbit stopped moving, I could see that a small section of skin around its neck was cut and had torn backwards, revealing a white underside of clean, shiny flesh, as if this part of its neck alone had been skinned. If the rabbit had remained very still, the skin might have fallen back into place, releasing it from the grip of the fence. But of course the rabbit couldn't sit still. It had struggled with increasing, mortal urgency against the tightening wire, so that this wire had cut into its neck. Beside the clean, white skin, its brown fur was matted with crimson blood which shone brightly in contrast to the dull tarnish of its eyes. I knelt down, very slowly. The rabbit quivered a little as it sensed my shadow over it. Then it pulled back against the wire again, inflicting further hurt on itself. And I saw, in this moment, that scrolling, scrolling, scrolling, scrolling, scrolling through my phone, looking for photos of her and at photos of her, as if by staring right at them I could make her death un-happen, I was the rabbit trying to resist the forwards pull of time.

Loss, I realized, was the shape of my sister and me since we were adolescents. And as I knelt, almost as if before that rabbit, I saw the images held in those photographs again. I had been searching for the images in which my sister looked straight back at me, since I felt that when I looked into her eyes I could trigger some kind of osmosis between her image and me. I'm not sure which direction I hoped the travel would be, but I felt as if by staring extremely hard at her either I could seep into the picture to join her there, or I could make her seep back to me. 'Seep' – the word still makes me think of her body underground and how it might be now and how the water and wet and worms would be working on her skin and bones and cartilage and hair (do worms eat hair?). Then I could not stop thinking about her body underground in her blue dress with stars on it and I could not stop wondering about whether she was still golden, as she had been when I last saw her, and I felt as much panic as the rabbit before me. Unlike the rabbit, I kept very still.

The rabbit scrambled some more against the wire, and when I put my hand out to try to release the tightening knot on its neck, it pulled back so hard that its eyes bulged. The photographs had made me think again how close are the edges between life and death but, like the rabbit pulling and pulling against its own life, mortally wounding itself, I knew that looking back at the images, pulling against time, was hurting me so much because there was no channel to cross between those edges. I was wrong to think that looking at her photographs could keep a sense of her alive. She was dead. I had watched her die. I had held her hand – held her – as she had died. I had put my arms around her, pressed my face against her chest and cheeks, pressed my heart against her heart, loved myself into her as she had died and she had sweated into me as she had died. That was the only seeping that would ever occur between our physical bodies. And I realized, too, that although I had turned to her photographs for comfort, the more I stared at them, the more acutely I felt like that rabbit, wounding itself again and again in mortal terror. I had turned to her photographs to find her, and instead just trapped myself in a place of great pain that I needed to escape from, although I had no sense of how to do that. There was nothing I could do for the rabbit. It was going to die. Still, very gently, I released it.

In February, two months after my sister had died, I realized that the days of magical thinking were blotched by more obstinate, familiar emotions, like big brown blocks obscuring my vision. Boredom, regret, irritation. Also anger, rage and fury, which came up out of some place deep inside me, a place I had not felt until it showed itself to me in this new, specific feeling of hatred for the fact of my sister's death. Sometimes, when I was standing at the school gate in the wind and the rain, holding a nylon book bag, I thought I could see her figure, in silver-blue or watery green satin (remember, she was a circus proprietor, so to see her dressed in green satin and ostrich feathers was to see her at work), vanishing way, way beyond my sight and I had to just fold the rage up flat and tuck it inside me so that it didn't cover everyone else at the school gates and stop them breathing too. I felt like a child excluded from an adult event I longed to be part of. Her union with death was regal, extreme, ecclesiastical. The route my life was taking was domestic, dull, monotonous, the stuff of the school gate, the inside of my car. Day followed day. I spent my time moving piles of toys the children had left in the kitchen, slapping cheese down a grater to shove into a white sauce, taking my anger at death out on the inside of the washing machine as I ripped clothes from the drum. There is nothing ancient or mystical about domestic life even when it comes slap bang up against the face of death. Domestic life just continues, even when what you really want to do is bury yourself alive with a chariot and all your favourite slaves, or send a burning ship out into the middle of an ocean. I longed to feel transformed by death. But just because we survive when the person we love doesn't, there is no guarantee that we will become stronger, better, bigger versions of ourselves. There was no guarantee I could be as unflinching as Gawain as he knelt before the Green Knight.

I was jealous of my sister. At the moment that I was clearing the table or bleaching the sink or just walking dully along, she was fathoming how to cross the Styx. How could I be left gripping the peeling black plastic of my Fiat Punto steering wheel as Dash and Lester fought over who got to open the window, while she was adventuring onwards in green silk and ostrich feathers? Time had become my arch-enemy, moving me towards each present moment, which is, of course, the future, so that the past – that moment where she was standing in front of me breathing and arguing and laughing – vanished, vanished, vanished, vanished, vanished,

*

I should confess to you, too, that I was fearful. I was extremely scared of depression. I did not want to slide into that nether world. Rage, at least, was hot and crackling and allowed me to check in with all my emotions. I'd been depressed, many times, when my sister was alive, and since clambering out of *that* pit had taken months and months of hard work, then how the fuck would I ever manage it when my sister was dead? If depression got me now, the children would be abandoned at the school gate and the washing would go mouldy in the machine and our dog and cat and horse would die from starvation and Pete – oh, I don't want to think about what it would be like for Pete if I went back into that pit.

Since I could not bear the pain of making my brain comprehend the reality that my sister was dead, I tried to take my brain away from her and what the loss of her meant altogether. Give it a sabbatical from death, if you like. I knew I couldn't make her death un-happen, but for a bit I tried something else: I put her and death into a small cupboard in my mind. I squashed them both into the smallest possible space, and leant on the door to shut and bolt them away. I visualized doing this in the way I did it in real life with the blankets and sleeping bags that spilled out of the cupboard on the upstairs landing. They were all much too big for the cupboard and I was too messy and lazy to fold them properly, but I am also strong and so if I leant against the cupboard I could easily shut the small gold catch on the door so that those blankets and sleeping bags were all contained there. I could dust my hands off and walk away.

There. See? I could walk up and down the landing now

and the blankets and sleeping bags, and my sister and her death, did not spill out on top of me. They were locked away in a place where I couldn't see the mess and confusion they made, so it didn't bother me. There were lots of little tricks my mind played on me and I played on it in order to manage death. There were whole moments and even entire hours when this worked for me in the later weeks after her funeral. When the heavy stone of death was not on string around my neck. I could pretend to myself, then, that death was not something I had met and must acquaint myself with and hold with me. This feeling of liberation from death was strongest when I woke up. The knights and the dark green forest had disappeared. I could even be very happy when I woke up. Hard white winter light would fall on the green walls of my bedroom and I'd be aware of the bedroom around me, the warmth of my heavy blankets, the feeling of a child nestled beside me. I felt safe to be awake and safe to find myself in a human life. But, then when I was properly awake, this sense of happy vanished and I was pulled out of the sweet, comfortable life I'd woken up in and back into the cold terrifying one in which death had visited and taken my sister away.

Back.

That was where I wanted to be.
  I wanted to go back.
  Back back back.

*

And there was one way I could get back. Dreams. In my dreams I found the people I needed to answer questions I couldn't ask in real life. Because if I asked my friends, 'How do I live now?' they didn't know the answers. Actually, that's not true: two of them did have answers. They are called Liz and Liv. Liz, whose wife had died, said, 'Surrender. Kneel down and surrender before death because it will always win and understanding that will make your life easier,' and Liv, whose mother had died, said, 'I promise you it will change and it will get easier when it does.' But other people still said, 'I cannot imagine what you are going through,' or, 'I imagine it's going to be very difficult for a long time for you,' or, 'You are doing so well.' This last phrase confused me the most. What was this thing that they were referring to that I was *doing* well?

One friend said to me that I had had so much loss in my life that if I could get through the year without killing myself I would be doing well. That took me aback a bit. Even I thought: Steady on!

But in dreams, when I saw people who I had thought were dead, I found they told me things that felt like pure truths. And when I dreamed of my sister, I became aware of my waking and sleeping worlds becoming the same space. My dreams were always full of a sense of anticipation of the pain I would find myself in when I woke up. When I first dreamed about her, it was as if we were both ten years younger, but in the dream, she knew she was going to die, and in this way the past and present, dream and real life, seemed to become one.

'They told me I had more time,' she said to me, and there was something accusatory in her voice, although I know she was not blaming me. (She was also articulating something I felt towards her doctor too – reproach – for he had indeed told us she had more time.)

In my dream I was worrying about the thought of losing her. 'They told me I had more time,' she repeated, and I knew I should help her. And also in the dream I was so afraid of the pain which lay ahead for her and for all of us in her inevitable death that it became a nightmare. And then I woke up and realized I was in that place I had been scared of in my dream. I was awake again and there was absolutely no way of being able to reach my sister. My face was wet, although it was also dawn, and the light from outside was golden yellow.

The dreams of my sister didn't happen as often as I would have liked them to, because I loved them, however much they disturbed me. But then one night, quite close to dawn, I became aware of being in the presence of a man called Dagir. I have written about him before, but I gave him a different name then as he was still alive, and he had said to me, 'My life very criminal, Clover, don't write of me.'

But he died two years before my sister, and although I had not seen him for eight years, the thought he was not alive somewhere in the world made me cry a lot. Because, although I would never have actually done it, since I love Pete with all my heart, when Dagir was alive there was always the possibility I could go and find him. I had been

in love with him and I'd also been in love with his land, as
he had. He was from Ossetia, in the Caucasus Mountains.
Even just thinking of the world he showed me – of mountains and black horses and men always in leather coats
with guns in their inside pockets or Kalashnikovs under
their car seats, of mountain huts and little girls sorting piles
of herbs alongside a pistol in abundant markets and of loss
and passion and melancholy – makes me feel alert and
acutely engaged. His death robbed me of a parallel world.
I will not go there again. It would hurt too much and be too
dangerous to attempt it without the close local protection
of those men with a gun always ready in their leather coats.

Now Dagir was standing in my room and I'm not even
sure this experience of seeing him again was a dream. It felt
different. He used to have a red T-shirt with Осéтия printed
on it, which means 'Ossetia', and the last time I saw him
wearing it was when we were riding through the Caucasus
Mountains. Then he had had a gun on his saddle and a leather bag with some herbs and some slices of cold meat in
it – I think it was lamb we'd cooked on a fire the day before,
and some vodka and small silver cups. (He died of alcohol-
ism, but these silver cups mattered since, unlike me, he
would absolutely never, ever drink vodka straight out of a
bottle.) In this non-dream that did, nonetheless, happen
while I was in a state of minimal consciousness, if not actually asleep, he was wearing the same red T-shirt and his
short black hair was very glossy. These physical details
were vivid, like the way he held his cigarette tight between

thumb and forefinger as he laughed at me, wiping away tears that were running down my cheeks.

'Do not cry,' he said, and then, smoking and laughing more, he pressed his strong thumbs too hard into my face, as he always had done, at Vladikavkaz Airport when I was saying goodbye to him. He had very strong hands in real life with which he touched my body all over, because I had really liked being held by him, and I was struck, at that moment and also after it, later in the morning, by his strong physicality, which was an important part of how I saw him in this dream. There was nothing spiritual or anything less than very substantial about him in this dream. There was nothing vague about him. He was physically there, almost close enough to fuck.

'I am not dead. Tamerlan got the dates wrong. When he called and told you I had died, he was wrong. I am not dead.' Everything around me tasted of tears and tobacco. Now we were sitting on green grass, as we often had been in England when I met him and then again in Russia when I went to see him. I met him in the circus and we were always sitting outside on the grass, often at night. When I looked down in the dream there was a child with him, a little girl with dark hair and dark eyes like his, her straight hair divided into pigtails, her pale skin glowing and white, precious pearl. He had some green and very glossy olives, which was characteristic of him. When I was with him in the circus and in Russia, he liked eating food outdoors, and had an ability to transform some slices of salami and pieces of bread and salt and a boiled egg and vodka into a marvellous occasion. In the circus, we often used to bang on my sister's door after the show was finished to ask her if she wanted to go for a picnic. No, she would say, she didn't want to go for a fucking picnic. She wanted to sit in a restaurant and drink champagne. Afterwards he always would laugh at night-time and say, 'Let's go for a fucking picnic,' and that's where I found myself with him in my dream, at a fucking picnic.

When I came around from this sleeping/dream/subconscious state I felt extremely excited and relieved. I had seen Dagir again. I had actually felt myself in his presence. He had been there with me and at that moment I was absolutely convinced I would see him again. He had shown me that sign and I was so grateful to him, because if he was still real, in another place, then that meant my sister was real, somewhere else, too.

Since I was trying to feel normal, and pretending to myself and other people that I was normal, in February half-term I chose to go to Devon to stay in the house of some friends who invited me there. I thought I would tell death to fuck off by choosing a wet weekend in a coastal town where even the local fish-and-chip bar had shut down, and all the toilet paper had run out in the one open tea-room. There couldn't be anything less heroic or epic than that, and I told myself that in those circumstances I wouldn't have to think about death. Death, after all, was reserved for the very, very special ones, the ones in watery green silk. Death, in its majesty, wasn't there for someone like me, with my stupid human responses and my stupid human hunger. Death didn't care if there were chips available or not. Death did not bother itself with things like toilet paper, or whether the car might run out of petrol on an especially busy stretch of the A303. Death was never concerned with all the prosaic stuff that was cluttering my life, while my sister became more essential and elemental and eternal.

It occurred to me, as I unpacked bags in the holiday house, regretting immediately I wasn't at home, that I would have felt more comfortable and secure in what was required of me if there had been another funeral to organize. If I could be allowed to organize my sister's funeral every two weeks for the rest of the year, my mind might be able to relax and find the safe space of serious ritual it was hunting for. The funeral had provided scaffolding that I could use to hold myself up in the weeks after she died. Obviously – OBVIOUSLY – I could not organize my sister's funeral every fortnight for a year, so instead I put my considerable will towards living NORMAL LIFE.

But then I found that other people around me didn't want me to be normal. Occasionally this made me want to smash a cup, I felt so angry about it and what death had done to me. From the other side of the doors in the holiday house in Devon I'd hear my friends laughing about a joke, and then when I came into the room the laughter would suddenly stop and they'd look solemn. At other times they'd rub my shoulder as they passed me sitting at the kitchen table, as if I too was really ill, as my sister had been. I felt impatient. I felt as if everyone was pretending around me and I wanted to shout at them to do something different, I wasn't sure what, but to stop pretending. I wanted to be like them: carefree, able to bake and ice a carrot cake, keen to sit up late and drink red wine, keeping death at a long arm's length, as they did.

I tried to compensate, taking my children down to the dark yellow sands where we laid out green strings of seaweed and dug sticks into the sand spelling out I LOVE YOU to each other, and also to her. There was a small beach cafe where I bought each child a stack of pancakes as we walked down to the beach, and again, on the way back. Such a treat! So many pancakes! The children covered them in caramel ice cream and golden syrup, spooning them into their little mouths until they rubbed their lips, telling me their teeth ached.

Did I really think that sugar and pancakes would make the pain go away, bring her back or stop me feeling lonely on holiday with my friends?

In Devon the sky whipped up above me, epic sunlight pouring down from the heavens, beckoning me with white light which talked to me, whispering that if I believed then here, out above the ancient oceans, might be where I'd find my sister. But I wanted to stop looking. Because I had looked and looked and looked. I had tried to see my dead sister in many other big skies, and bright orange satsumas, and green flashing eyes of jet-black cats. I'd pounced on these signs and held them so close to me, frantic that they might show me how to find my sister and, crucially, how to hold on to an actual physical, irrefutable signal that she had not gone. But I was sick of the signs. I knew they were all lies, or not real, because nobody – NOBODY – could claim she was anywhere nearby now.

So I ignored the big exciting skies and the magical signs and in defiance I thought instead about cottage pie, which needed making for supper, playing cards, since I wanted to teach my children how to play 21, and tobacco, as I'd started smoking again. Holding a cigarette in my fingers at the end of my arm was possibly as fun and exciting as I knew how to be. And it was a little dangerous, not because of the heart disease and lung cancer it might bring with it, but because it meant I had to leave the house and stand outside on my own, which made me think hard. And of course, when you smoke, you naturally look upwards, or outwards, and then the mind starts searching and imagining again.

'Stop being so fucking stupid,' I told myself aloud when two grey clouds parted beside the full moon to reveal a single star, just at the moment that I was thinking about her. 'It's just a star.' And then to distract myself as I smoked a second cigarette, I looked up what a star was made of on my phone, which I was clutching, of course. And a star, I read, is nothing more than a luminous mass of hydrogen and helium, with nuclear fusions in its core which support it against gravity and produce photons and heat. It's a physical part of the universe which scientists can explain, although a definition of astronomy on a webpage also told me, as I scrolled in the cold, that 'historically the most prominent stars were grouped in constellations and asterisms, the brightest of which gained proper names'. I let my mind rest and bathe in the ethereal glittery beauty of the noun *constellation*. And skipping through the science, on the screen I focused on words like *stellar nucleosynthesis* and *supernova* and *celestial luminosity*, which all sounded like the kind of environments that my sister might well inhabit.

But the effect of this was that when I ground the end of my cigarette into the wet moss outside the house, and went back inside where the long table was laid for supper, I could not make my brain think about cottage pie. My brain kept skipping back into the night, dying to go up there with the stars, where it really wanted to be, and so then, rather than standing upright, I had a *gravitational collapse*.

I was relieved to go home after that, but I was still looking for times when I could let my mind focus on something other than my sister. Almost three months after her death, I had to go to London for two days, one after the other, for my work. I had avoided working for the whole of December and January but, by February, that wasn't possible any more. And I found I wanted to immerse myself in it. I imagined it might be a good place to be, focusing on my keyboard rather than focusing on the loss. I had to create a new kind of normality, and work might be a way of forging that.

Pete drove me to the station at Didcot Parkway. The

radio was on in the car and we talked about normal things that were happening that week, like the children's parents' evening and a meeting Pete had which meant he might have to go to Brussels and whether the MOT was due on the car. On the radio, there was a report on the virus that was spreading from Italy, but it seemed very distant, so I ignored it and talked to Pete. I felt calm in his presence, so I didn't tell him that I felt as if my life was over, or that I didn't know how to feel comfortable with my existence, and that instead I was thinking of myself as a kind of sacrifice given up when my sister died. This was much, much easier than trying to feel happy and I could exist in that place quietly. I felt quite accepting of this. There was no need to tell anyone. I would be able, I felt, to go through the rest of my life just talking and stepping through the days, even if the reality I was existing inside was this strange and empty place where there would never really be joy again, and light would always be like shaded dusk, or if it was dawn, so fucking beautiful it was too poignant even to look straight at. I had an absolute sense of sitting in the passenger's seat as Pete drove and, for the first time in my adult life, feeling like a total passenger. I could laugh occasionally, but there was always this sense of the petrol-blue presence of death sitting on my shoulder like a jackdaw.

Pete sat carefully beside me on the train all the way to London and held my hand without letting go, as though I was a small, empty doll. I was relieved for him that he could not see the anger like upturned nails which suddenly pierced something inside me whenever the memory that she was dead and I would never see her again came over me. In order to suppress it, I stared very hard out of the window. I remember a heap of small wooden rowing boats, piled up like coffins in a muddy field near Reading. The flat dark light on the river was a colour I'd never seen before and didn't know the name for, so I tried to describe the colour of it to myself to quieten the rage inside me.

I had to go to an office near Tottenham Court Road, and Pete walked me to the taxi rank. He put his hands around my face and squeezed me a bit as he does to make me feel myself, but I was not really there. I had disassociated from my life. I was the opposite of bold or wild and sleepless or chivalric. Just absent. So Pete put me into a taxi. As the car drove off I watched the grey edges of the city pass in a blur outside the window, but as the cab stopped, the driver asked me if I was OK, which startled me, as I'd forgotten I was visible.

'You look, well, a bit lost.'

I wanted to tell him about this rage I felt because of my dead sister but instead I just lied: 'Fine, thanks, I'm fine.'

'Well, have a wonderful day,' he said. I watched the black of his cab vanishing down the street and had a powerful urge to run after him, rap on his window with my knuckles and ask him for instructions: *A wonderful day? What do you mean? What is that? How do I get that?*

I had to go into a meeting for an hour to talk about something new I might be writing. I was very aware, from the softness in her voice to the searching way she looked at me, that the woman I had gone to see was making an extra effort to be kind to me. And for that time, probably less than an hour, I felt as if all the other things that were happening in my life – the big and difficult feelings – were absent. For a few moments, I was the person I had been before death got close to me. But then the meeting finished, and I had to walk back outside, so unstable, alone, trying to navigate my way as if blind with arms outstretched. Except that when I came out on to the pavement, I noticed a row of yellow chairs which I had not seen as I'd walked in. They were piled up in high stacks and the brightness of them looked sort of stunning. How bright and beautiful they were, I thought, like the blackbird I could suddenly hear, singing, as I walked to meet a friend who had been at my sister's funeral. We went to a ramen cafe and I knew we would have to talk about my sister's funeral although I didn't really want to.

'It was all so close,' I said to my friend. 'I can't remember it. It was too close to remember it.'

He looked at me with eyes that seemed as if they might cry. 'It's OK not to remember it.' He had not yet eaten anything but now put his spoon back into his bowl of ramen. 'It's more than OK not to be able to remember the funeral. You *were* it.'

I didn't know what to say so I pressed my hand against my forehead so that I could feel the outer edges of myself. Everything around me felt too loud in my ears and unbelievably close to my face. I could see so many faces leaning forward, slurping bowls of ramen, and some of them laughing as they ate. It seemed all wrong. I didn't understand how all the people could be eating ramen. Had they gone on eating ramen all through December at the moment that my sister had been dying?

Later, I took the train back to Didcot on my own as Pete had had to stay in London, so he was not there to hold my hand. I missed the fast train because I had been mesmerized by a video playing on a screen in a hotel in Paddington where I'd stopped to use the toilet. It was in the bar, where men in suits were sitting in front of laptops and a woman in a long purple tweed jacket was having a loud conversation on her mobile about seeing her mother that weekend and how expensive a return to Manchester was. All of these people were ignoring the screen behind them, where a supermodel in a floor-length red dress repeatedly walked towards them, swirling around just as she reached a point where she seemed almost close enough to touch. THE GAZE IS REAWAKENED, the screen read, although no one in the bar apart from me seemed to be gazing, let alone feeling anywhere close to being reawakened by it. I felt as if everything was there for me as messages that I was supposed to be able to understand, although actually knowing how to decipher those messages was apparently impossible. And I started wondering if death might illuminate everyone who touches it into something bigger and brighter and redder, so that for a moment it could make us all feel like supermodels in red sequinned dresses. And I remembered, too, my sister, a long time ago, standing in the snow in a red satin dress, and I made that strange gasping noise. The noise was what I was feeling inside: a physical, lurching longing to go back there, to the snow and the night when we were teenagers together. Thinking about my sister felt like two crystals touching and at that moment I understood I was learning about pain. And I realized the longer my training in pain, the deeper and more true my understanding of it would be.

But I still could not stop thinking about the physical shape that death must take. Because this was the thing. I had been in the room with death. On the top floor of the hospital I had been right inside the room with death; it had stood quietly beside my sister and me in the last few hours, just waiting to do its thing. My sense of death arriving in that hospital ward had been so strong. The pressing down from above of the petrol-blue wings which took everyone's breath from the room, squeezing the breath out as it wrapped itself about my sister and folded those wings around her and took her.

Thinking about this made me cry and when I tasted salt on my lips I thought that, like Lot's wife, I was looking back, and sometimes that made me feel that existing as a pillar of salt would have been preferable to all this scarlet, bloody human feeling which made my blood so terribly bright. I watched that last day of my sister's life in my head all the time, wanting more than anything to make her life happen again. And while it pressed over her, this huge, huge presence of death turned me into something very small and screwed-up, like a piece of paper with biro scribbles all over it that means nothing. I wanted to hear her voice. I wanted to know where she was. I couldn't hear her voice and when I thought about the fact I'd never hear her voice talking to me again, I wanted to scream and scream and scream until I broke my own voice into nothing.

Nine weeks after she died I went to her house, before it was cleared, to sort her clothes and organize her most personal possessions for her children. Her house was to be rented out. Someone's home holds them for a while after they die. Walking into my sister's big dining room, where a long table filled the room, and seeing her easel set up where she had been painting a bull, I felt like part of her being was still and frozen in the air there. Her house was filled with art and objects that had been part of her circus, but which now felt dead. There were tapestries, costumes, sketch books, flags, masks, embroideries, but also all her paintings, which she had created almost incessantly in the last years of her life. In her rooms were easels and plates with paint still on them in coloured dots where she had mixed them: reds and greens, blue, yellow, purple, as if multicoloured tears had spilled there.

But I was there to sort things out. I was going to meet my father and my stepmother and we would *sort things out*. I felt breathless: I was to look right into the physical being of my sister's life and I felt like a diver about to step off the outside of a boat. When I arrived at her house my dad and stepmother were there already. Both of them were dressed in black. They were looking nervous, as if their hearts had been opened up.

'Clove, Clove,' my dad said, patting my back as he hugged me, the front door still open behind us. I was more aware than I have ever been before that I was standing in front of the man who was my sister's father. He was a part of her, as I was. I was aware, too, of the missing person, even more than I had been for several weeks. My father's eyes had changed since my sister had died. My stepmother hugged me; her cheeks were warm, but we all had a wide-open look. We were all divers: I could see that.

For a bit, we walked through the house, room to room. The inside of my mind felt like a tuning fork that had been tapped and was vibrating, alone, trying to find the right note. I was aware, too, that things were changing almost in front of my eyes. Immediately after she died, in the days when I went to her house to meet with other family members, it was as if some of her things, like her coats, her books, a plate with her name on, had actually contained an essence of her. At that point, straight after death, she had left part of herself on everything. At the time I had thought that by holding her things, I could feel closer to her.

Now I walked through her house and looked again, two months later, for those same imprints of her. Her riding boots, black leather, were standing by the front door, an imprint of sawdust on one of them, as if she might step back into them right away. There was her mackintosh, and when I lifted it up, the shapes of the arms were not flat, like a coat that had been hanging unworn, but contained her still. Her arms had been the last arms in the coat. I had held her arms as she lay dying. I had tried to press myself into every part of her as she lay in the hospital bed and I remembered how soft and warm her arms were. How strong she was.

I lifted it to my face, but the coat was waxed and smelt of cold outdoors, not of her. I pulled my arms into the place where her arms had been. I tried to imagine my sister inside it but instead I thought again of the stone knights in Gloucester Cathedral and I wondered if their sisters or mothers or lovers went and ran their hands over the stone arms that were left behind. I needed armour but I did not, at that moment, feel comfortable having my arms in the place her arms had been. I was quite sure she must be walking across the yard towards the house. She must be about to come back inside and it would not be right to be wearing her work coat when she arrived. I waited for her to come through the door, for the moment I could hug her, when her big cheekbone would touch mine, and our knowledge that we were made from the same stuff would be impossible to deny, even if we had been fighting over something quite recently.

But she didn't come in. She didn't come back, even though I waited, sure that by putting my arms into her coat I could make her return. When I turned back to the room, all I could hear was my father talking to my stepmother in another room and otherwise the house sounded empty. I couldn't hear my sister in her own house.

I tried to do the things she would have liked. I felt that by breaking up sticks to start a fire, striking a match from black to flame yellow and then lifting that flame to the paper in the stove, perhaps I could conjure up something of her. The paper flared up in the flame, sudden light and warmth, and there was a crackle of life as the twigs caught. I thought of her kneeling before the grate, pushing a log into her fire, and I realized that everything burns eventually. For a bit I sat back on my heels and waited, watching the flames work through the paper and take hold amongst the sticks. My sister had loved the smell of a fire when it mixed with toast. I left the door of the stove open, the flames moving inside there, and in the kitchen sliced two pieces of brown bread which I put into the toaster, turning the dial around to high, so that the toast would burn. Then I went back and sat in front of the stove again and watched the flames.

Being in her house made me feel two things: both exquisitely closer to her, surrounded by her books, her coats, her china, her green sofa and green sitting room, and also so lost to her that the feeling was like tight pressure around my throat. I felt sorry for her plants: geraniums, bright red, on every window ledge, straining against the inside of the windows as though they were waiting, waiting, waiting and might soon die with waiting.

My father and stepmother and I sat at her table and drank tea from her cups. A couple who had distantly known my sister arrived uninvited, offering help. The wife wore a pink polo shirt, neatly pressed, and he had on a blue tank top. I tried to concentrate on these colours as they talked. The woman nodded her blonde head and laughed and I thought that perhaps this was what it felt like to be deaf, or autistic: out of sync but also seeing the things that mattered.

'We could fill boxes for you,' they said but we shook our heads. The formality of having to have a conversation about what we were doing felt like a very heavy, pointless burden, Sisyphus pushing a rock up a hill over and over again. I wanted to be alone with my father and my step-mother to take up an important challenge – to stare death in the face as I held my dead sister's clothes – and not be talking with these stupid people who didn't seem to know things that would be useful: where the cupboard was where bin bags might be kept, or the times the charity shops shut. After they had gone, we all stared at one another and I heard us all breathing out. The kitchen smelt of wood smoke and burnt toast and when I looked at one of the geraniums on the window sill, I noticed it had shed red petals that moved, very slightly, as my father turned around and filled the kettle again, quickly, with iron-coloured water from the tap.

We drank more tea and then my stepmother and I went upstairs to sort out my sister's clothes. We did not say it, but I know neither of us wanted my father to have to do this. I kept thinking of the sound my father had made to express pain at my sister's bedside in the moments when she had died.

'I've got absolutely fuck all to wear,' my sister had said to me a few weeks before she was dead, with her real-life living voice. This was around about the time she had been told by her oncologist she could well live for another ten years. Now, though, my stepmother and I were stand-ing in her attic, sorting through racks and racks and racks of clothes: a green sequinned Gucci bomber jacket, a floor-length red Marni snakeskin coat, a black lace Chanel scarf, sky-high Alexander McQueen boots. If throwing money at the problem of life worked, the proof manifested itself in my sister's clothes.

In her room there was a fine layer of dust on the glass chest of drawers beside her bed. When she was alive, there would never have been dust there. When she was alive, her room would have sparkled.

I moved around the bedroom, putting my hands on her things. The jolting, almost electric shock of placing my hand on a book we had been talking about two months before. Heart-breaking, unopened wands of black mascara. The little bottles of lavender oil on the shelf. Her jewelled hair clip with a strand of hair attached. Pots of half-used face cream, a tub of coconut oil, the end of a can of dry shampoo and lots of almost finished bottles of bath oil.

I moved my hand across a red and black lumberjack coat from Isabel Marant which was hanging over the back of a chair.

'I think I look like a Canadian,' she'd said to me, two years before, as I stretched out on the armchair in her bedroom after she'd returned from Bicester Village. She was newly divorced then and had had new pale blue silk curtains made for her bedroom ('I thought I should make it a bit more glamorous') and a gas fire fitted that looked like a real fire except that it burned hard and consistently and never made any mess. ('You must get one. It's a game changer. Put one in your bedroom, Pete would love it.')

When I saw the coat, I remembered her frowning as she tried it on. 'Does it matter if I look like a Canadian? That I might be going to chop wood? I probably am going to chop wood.'

Now I had a sense that a monster or minotaur was with me, invisible but deadly present, standing quietly in a corridor upstairs, its breath misting the air, ready to roar and terrify just at the moment when I opened my sister's top drawer and found a little pile of black socks, folded together like sleeping kittens. It savaged me in her bathroom as I reached out and touched her toothbrush, her hairbrush with some of her bright blonde hairs in it, a neat little line of diamanté hair clips (always a dazzle and glitter around her, remember the circus) that she'd left there a few weeks before. It got hold of me and terrified me, beating me down so that I slid to her bathroom floor and allowed it to maul me. But my stepmother was there, and my father was downstairs, cooking a chicken pie, and although the monster or minotaur could work on them at any moment too, at least we were together, a version of Theseus. We all had a ball of string which was the life together that we shared, which we could hold on to to find our way out of the labyrinth and leave the minotaur standing alone in the dark, hot and dripping and breathing.

I realized that even up to as late as that moment, I had been trying somehow to pretend she wasn't dead. I had been falling into a state of confusion in order to allow my brain to swim around, like a bee in a puddle. But standing in her room, opening her drawers, finding carefully folded black T-shirts, pants, running shorts, I knew, absolutely, that I couldn't go on pretending she might not actually have gone, or that she might just have gone to the other side of the world for an imprecise amount of time. I couldn't go on pretending that she was coming back, or that I could go back. I thought suddenly of a conversation we had had, just a few months ago. She was talking about the idea of one day getting a flat in London so that she could leave the darkness and mud of the countryside and go to the city at will. That's the dream, she said. Remembering this I had to put one hand down to steady myself against her glass drawers, because I was ashamed that I should have the knowledge she never had, which was that she would die. That this flat in London would never happen and I would be standing in her bedroom amongst her old things, ready to pack them into cardboard boxes. My hand on the drawers where I'd pressed it to stop myself falling over left an imprint on the dust, as if someone else was touching my fingertips from inside the glass.

That night I lay in a bed in my sister's house. I was a bit drunk, since after we'd filled my sister's life into black plastic bags or airtight ziplock bags, my father and my stepmother and I sat at her table to eat the chicken pie and we drank some wine. Enough wine, in fact, to blunt the sharp edges of pain around us. The smell of burnt toast was gone and things had been moved around so that I no longer recognized where my sister had kept things. But the kitchen was still hers, in an intensely recognizable way: gold cups glistening in the kitchen cupboard, a map of Romania plastering the wall, her handwritten sign that read 'Please smoke' and a green and blue geometric cartoon of a train that had been in our father's study when we were growing up which I would later take from the wall and hang in my own house. We stayed up until it was late, talking together, and then I went to the double bed in my sister's spare room and lay still, listening for her. Time felt unstable and so did my relationship with death. It was becoming clearer that things like Devon and mashed potatoes and driving my car must all happen, of course – for sure they must happen – but that I also had this big task and I had to keep working on it. I had to learn more about my relationship with death, and also my relationship with my sister, now she was dead. I had thought I could use a wet week in Devon to move on to the next bit of my life. I had imagined my life as it had been before could start again but of course it could not. I felt so tired. The task ahead was huge and only I could fulfil it. I thought of a picture we had of a Pre-Raphaelite-looking woman with long red-golden hair, touching a knight on each of his shoulders with a long sharp sword. His head was bowed but he was ready to go out from the court and quest.

I saw myself now most clearly like the knight with the pointed silver blade lifted to his shoulders. I had to stop waking up and thinking she was alive. Other people had made this step, after all. The letters and emails that continued to arrive were from people who knew she was dead. Those people who wrote the letters did not, I now knew, wake up imagining my sister was still alive. It would take a magic trick for normal life to resume. A huge effort of will. Until then my mind had not been able to comprehend death, in the same way that my son Lester's mind could not comprehend a hundred. But it had to be done, again and again every time I woke up. And just as Lester had to learn maths to read the world, I had to learn about death to read my new world.

'Be careful, Clove!' my father called to me after we had hugged, saying goodbye. He patted me on my back again, and I pushed myself into the car alongside some of my sister's plants, three paintings, a jersey, some black shirts and a black dress that would otherwise have gone to a charity shop. Close to the ditch by the verge that ran alongside a strip of trees near my sister's house, a tree was split open, revealing a bright yellow-white colour inside its dark green-brown bark. It was appalling and almost prehistoric – the huge roots, upturned and ripped up, lying on their side, shockingly perpendicular to the firm footing in which that tree must have grown for a century. I didn't want to look at the destruction of it since it made me think of the fresh carcass of a dinosaur.

Instead, I thought about my driving because being in a car is a place where death feels close. I had lately become more aware of this and found traffic approaching from the right at a junction made me feel especially vulnerable. Strong flashes of the terrible sound of a car crash often came to mind. A part of me has become increasingly sure that I will die in a car; since the images arrive with me so strong and fast, I feel I already know what might happen. My sister lived on the edge of a deep valley, so driving took extra concentration there, and that day, after non-stop rain, there was water coursing down the hills. I drove to my friend's house; she had made lunch for me with her two brothers who live close by. She was also a friend of my sister, and she and one of her brothers had come to the hospital in the last few hours of my sister's life.

As I arrived, she was leaning out of an upstairs window waving, like a woman in an Italian film. Her house sits on the edge of a very steep hill so that if you start thinking or worrying about it too much, you can imagine it toppling off the edge. When she appeared before me she was wearing bright red lipstick and a tight blue knee-length velvet jacket over jeans and trainers. Her black hair was shining and cut very short. She had looked like this when I had turned around in the hospital corridor, in those last two days, and she had been there, putting her arms around me as I pressed my face into the darkness. Her presence was reassuring beyond measure since she understood, she was capable of feeling everything that was inside me at that moment. In the hospital her brother, broad and physically strong, reassuring in the same way she was, had been wearing a long cloak with a hood, bringing something both ecclesiastical and theatrical into the intense, unrelentingly sanitized corridors of the hospital ward. They had been there, fleetingly, fuzzily, at my sister's funeral but this was the first time I'd sat with them since moving into the new world in which my sister was absolutely dead.

I gave the brother one of the bright red potted geraniums I'd taken from my sister's house. He was friends with her: they used to take a picnic with plates in a hamper to the hill between their houses. I imagined that they had white napkins and a checked picnic blanket and probably proper glasses and knives and forks with heavy bone handles. I wanted him to tell me what she had been like with him on those picnics and what they had talked about.

'Mostly metaphysical poetry,' he replied, and I wondered if he noticed the little jolt that went through me, which made me return my fork to the plate before it had reached my mouth. 'We are both shy, though, and I am socially awkward, so there were a lot of silences, but being with her was always wonderful. I think she was socially awkward too.' He smiled remembering this but he looked sad when he talked about my sister and I thought that this was because her death was now much more present than her life was.

There was a heavy tapestry on one wall behind the long table where we were eating lunch and a mannequin wearing a red tailored jacket with very big silver buttons stood beside the table as though it might wait on us if we just willed it hard enough. My friend and her two brothers smoked incessantly even as we ate, laughing as they talked over one another, red wine glinting like darkened blood in glasses, a huge joint of beef, red in the middle, on the table, surrounded by that chain of cigarettes and smoke. Another woman was there for lunch too. She was wearing a neat floral dress with pearl buttons and she asked me polite questions about the book I was writing and where I lived. I could barely see her through the cigarette smoke but it was nice to witness life in soft focus for a bit and after a while I picked up a cigarette from one of the three packets on the table and smoked too.

My friend and her brothers have experienced so much sudden and untimely death in their lives that at that moment, having been so close to it myself, I could feel that it was present in the way they communicated with one another. They all spoke over each other and often seemed to be speaking in riddles. They talked freely about a meal that had been cooked the night before a death, all remembering suddenly the humour of that evening although death had rushed into their house the following day. Sitting at their table as I listened to them remembering someone else who had died whom they all loved, I was aware that when we come close to and really confront death we see a version of life at its most compassionate and most generous and also most kind. That gave me a sense that a familiarity with death could be very beautiful. I felt no shame showing my friend and her brothers my weakness and pain when I was talking about my sister and my voice suddenly cracked in that way which can be embarrassing. I felt only relief to be with them and experience the sense they gave me of becoming part of a huge, endless group of other humans putting their faith in one another and showing their weakness.

'In the hospital, seeing you all,' my friend said, her voice trailing off for a moment as she pushed her plate away and pulled another cigarette from a packet, 'we were united in loss. Your family has lived through a great deal of loss. But . . .' She paused for a moment, gesturing to a further horizon, beyond the windows. '. . . your loss of your sister, your personal loss of your sister, who we all loved, of course we all loved, but still, *your sister*, is a different kind of loss, since her death severs you from your shared childhood. She's the person who you shared your earliest experience of being a human with. It's the shared childhood and the toys and books and your ponies, but also the shared emotions that have made you both who you are – sadness and joy, patience and rage. Shared survival. And now in the loss of your sister maybe you feel broken in half, as if a symmetry is broken, although I don't think it will always be gone. You will be yearning for a long time for her but maybe not forever. Maybe you will find something of her in your own life.'

Death brings out the love that's part of being human, I thought, as they all went on talking, remembering their dead friends, the sound of their overlapping voices interrupted by the clash of a tarnished silver fork dropped on a plate, more laughter and the glug of crimson fluid into glasses. I felt wiped in their tears but also very much alive, and safe with them: I could exist within my pain because it was a room they sat in too. I was aware of watching them, since we now shared this room together, trying to work out how they had done it. I couldn't start doing close interviews with them all, making notes on my phone, but if I could, I would have done. They could live with death and still cook roast beef and laugh and have their friends around a table and talk about good things that had happened both in the recent and long-distant past. They did not seem to be biding their time until death. I had felt that my life now would be a silent waiting game, but being with my friends that day showed me that if I studied, and came to understand the paths that they walked, there could be another kind of life following death I could live.

Chapter 4

The Century of a
New Kind of Destruction

One morning in mid-February, to make myself do something, to press onwards towards an unknown future as
Gawain had done, I left Dash and Lester with Pete and
drove to the riverbank about twenty minutes away from our
home with Evangeline. For the past four summers, my sister
and I had met regularly at this stretch of the river to swim,
or sometimes not to swim, but to just lie there with a picnic
or just to meet to talk. As I walked to the edge of the river
across the field of cows, I thought of the last time I had
been there with her at the end of the previous summer. We
both had red swimming suits to change into and we arrived
at lunchtime and didn't leave until it got dark. Dash had
brought a lot of train track with him to play with and my
sister's children and my children were together on the

banks with both their mothers. My sister had made lamb sandwiches and brought some plastic boxes of chopped up peppers and carrots. After a while we lit a fire. Our sauce-pan wasn't big enough to boil enough water, though, and as it was clear we were going to spend the rest of the day by the river, it was so hot and still, I left my children with my sister and drove quickly into the little town near the river and found a charity shop where I bought a tarnished gold kettle with its lid missing. We boiled water and sat beside the river all afternoon, with the sound of the chil-dren around us and a swan moving almost silently through the dark river. Afterwards we told one another it had been one of the best afternoons of our entire lives.

'Let's go again soon. Let's do that lots more times,' we said to each other.

If someone had said to me that afternoon that it would be the last time I would swim in that stretch of river with my sister, I would not have believed them. I know I would have slapped them or done some kind of violence to them for saying such a terrible and unthinkable thing.

I tried to both think about this and not think about it as I walked across the field with Evangeline, who was talking to me at the same time about a maths test. I didn't want to get into the river but I also felt compelled to get into the river, even though it was February, in order to plunge my body into a different state. I thought of Gawain riding towards a green castle where there was a huge green knight with a green horse and green skin and green armour. I wore the same red swimming costume I'd worn when I swam with my sister, and as I stood on a towel that squelched into the mud, taking my clothes off, shivering, with another towel wrapped over my shoulders, I could feel Evangeline watching me and making funny faces. She was wearing a beret which was decorated with a leopardskin print and a long gold puffa jacket that was mine and which I had wrapped around her to keep her warm. I felt she might be looking at me in the same way I had once looked at my mother when she swam in a Scottish lake in August and I had refused to get in. I had to move very quickly so as not to lose my drive forward into the water. There was more mud on the bank I had to walk through but I stepped fast into the water and when I was in it was like black blades all around me. It was terrifyingly cold and it gave me a deep and primal sense that death could be anywhere. It could be there, in the pain and the iron coldness of the water. But at the same time, it also made me feel deeply alive. This was the same stretch of water my sister and I had swum in so maybe the same water had been around her body when she swam. I thought about something my sister had told me once, that all the water in the world was the same water that had always existed even when the dinosaurs and the Ice Age were here and that there was no new water anywhere. So it was also possible that the same water which ran deep underground through her body was now surrounding me too.

I made myself take five big strokes but as I did so I felt myself cry from very deep inside me because the water was icy and so black. I could think about nothing except that exact moment, my mind concentrated into a hard single place where no doubt or fear or uncertainty could take hold. Afterwards it was as if those seconds might have been a long time.

Evangeline didn't understand what I was doing and neither did I, but I felt different in a better way when I scrambled back on to the bank. My whole body was shaking and juddering as I peeled my black socks back on. I worried that it was another of those moments when I was scaring Evangeline by behaviour that was too extreme for a mother. I could feel her small face still watching me intently as we bundled back into the car and I turned the heat up. What she really wanted, more than anything, was for me to take her to a cafe we'd passed on the way. That was her heart's desire.

Inside the cafe I was more aware than I should have been of the sound of a china cup hitting a saucer and the scrape of a chair across the wooden floor but it was reassuring to feel Evangeline's small hand holding mine as we waited for her drink. Her cup looked too big for her as she sat across the table from me, but the marshmallows bobbed around in it when she stirred it and I could sense her pleasure in her hot chocolate drink and I decided to just concentrate on that. She was talking to me about school and a project she had been doing on bats. I was trying to make myself focus on her face and her teeth, white inside her mouth, as she was speaking, since at the same time I was remembering my sister's face, when she was talking to me on the final day of our lives together. Her face, like Evangeline's, was unlined, expectant. Watching Evangeline, and nodding at her as she talked and cups clinked loudly on saucers all around me, I kept remembering the undisturbed but vulnerable look on my sister's face and I wondered what she'd seen as she looked beyond us while we were talking that last time. I thought of a veil lifting or perhaps a veil so translucent she could see through it. What did she see? On the side of Evangeline's saucer was a long, long teaspoon lying at an odd angle and I stared at it while still smiling to try to stop myself from crying. My sister and I used to have a word for objects that were strange-looking, awkward or lying at odd angles. We called them 'nosy'. Only she would have known that that long, long teaspoon was nosy. No one else would ever understand that. Evangeline kept talking to me and smiling and her white teeth flashed in her pink mouth.

Later, on the last stretch of road before the house, two deer crossed in front of the car.

Was that her saying, *I am here*?

That was her saying, *I am here*.

Everyone was now talking about the virus in Wuhan that seemed to be moving forwards, outwards, although we were all still blind to what was happening. No one wanted to look at death in the form of a virus flying around the world. No one wants to look at death in any form, ever.

But it was whirling around in late February – still at a distance, but making everything feel very different. I wanted to talk to my sister about it. She loved anything that was extreme and part of her was always primed for an apocalypse. When

Isis first appeared on the daily news she talked about it often. 'What would you do, what would you do, for example, if Isis just took over everything? What would you do if there was suddenly a massive civil war? Where would you go and what would you do?'

Death had deprived the pair of us of some extremely interesting and definitely funny conversations about stock-piling and self-sufficiency, I thought, as I watched Jimmy and his friend Teyte digging up our neglected vegetable patch in one corner of the garden and the radio in the kit-chen informed me that rationing might start. (Once, a few months before she died, we had been talking about general disarray in government, and she said that politics was like the new box set: she just wanted to watch the news all the time. She also said, 'And can't Jimmy do something? Kick off a rave as a big protest or something? Like we did in the nineties?')

But now I could not talk to her about these things and I felt very, very angry about that, but I was also preoccupied by other things that suddenly felt very different too. My hands, for one thing. They hurt like hell, dried by soap and water, and by the amount of time I was now spending hold-ing Dash and Lester's palms under the tap, while they sang 'Happy Birthday' (twice) to anyone they knew, which was how long we were supposed to clean ourselves for, to remove the virus from our hands. There was a new unease: a constant, twitchy worry, a tightening we all felt as we went about our lives. Everyone was looking away from death, or perhaps looking at it from the corners of their eyes. The virus was now in Lombardy and the videos from hospital wards in Italy were harder to look away from or pretend they were so far away as to not be a problem. I could see that people do this with death. I had done this with death for the previous five years, since the autumn of 2015 when my sister was first diagnosed. We had all looked away because visualizing the exact thing we were living through was too frightening. Pretend it's not part of our lives when it's actually everything and it's everywhere and it's going to happen any time. That's what death makes people do.

In late February the old life of normal shops, open schools, cafes and packed trains was still in full swing. Because the children were occupied in school I went to write in a coffee shop in a small town near our home. As I sat there a man came in. He was wearing a very formal suit and tie, the kind of old-fashioned suit I think I can remember a lot more people wearing when I was a child. He was with a much younger man, who steered him through the coffee shop to a table near mine, in the window. The younger man had a small backpack over one shoulder with the zip half undone as if he'd left in a hurry and he was wearing an almost luminous yellow anorak. His glasses were slightly wonky, as if knocked askew in the effort of helping the older man (who I felt must be his grandfather because of a shared countenance) into the right seat safely. The younger man was tender with him, patiently waiting while he fumbled over the hot-drinks menu, choosing several different elaborate types of coffee before settling on a cup of tea with no milk. Then the younger man went to the till to order it and I sat there just bathing in my computer light while actually watching this old-fashioned-looking man. Afterwards they sat at their table sharing a millionaire's shortbread and their conversation ranged on to what was actually happening in the world. The younger man was carefully explaining that coffee shops like this might have to close.

'It may be for a few days or perhaps as long as two weeks,' said the younger man, who had straightened his glasses now and was leaning forward to drink coffee from his big white cup the size of a bowl.

'Why are the shops closing? Are all shops closing?' The older man looked confused and by his stance I could see the younger man felt uncomfortable. He didn't know how much of this new idea of death to talk about with the older man.

'Well, the reason is there's a virus about,' he said quickly, suddenly sitting up straight and wiping shortbread crumbs from the table neatly into his palm, then depositing them like loose sand on to his saucer.

'Like a cold?' said the older man.

'Yes, like a cold,' the younger man replied, leaning forward again and folding his arms in front of him on the table. 'Like a cold. But it's killing people.'

'How does it do that?' said the older man, looking suddenly affronted, as if he had been told he was trespassing. The younger man looked down at his feet, then up once more.

'No one's quite sure. But it increases the chances of death.' Then he looked away, and down at his watch.

Wouldn't it be funny, I thought, snapping my laptop shut, splashing oat milk latte on to the table in front of me, if we could decrease the chance of death down to nothing? Why do we all walk around pretending that the fact we are alive means there is no chance of death? I thought about these things as I walked back to my car and unlocked the door, dumping my laptop bag in the footwell and belting myself in.

Blondie was playing on the radio as I drove home, and I knew I was pressing the accelerator too hard but I couldn't help it. It made me feel light and easy in a way I hadn't for ages. It made me think I might just vanish and that was a relief. Sometimes when I'm having sex I think of a car crash to make myself come; maybe this is part of the thing I have inside me that makes me prefer sex when it's violent. This makes me think that death excites me since I am fantasizing about the moment I will die. I imagine the sound the metal and glass and bone will make slamming together, and I wonder where the blood will go and the colour it will be.

As I pulled into the drive, Pete came out to the car to talk to me. He said he would probably have to close his office in London. He told me he'd heard reports that students were being called up to dig mass graves. I shook my head, because I didn't know what to say to him. The world turned, and it was more strange and unreadable than ever.

Later, when I was reading to Dash and Lester while thinking about other things, I remembered a joke, if you can call it that, which my sister and I sometimes shared, if we touched, tentatively, on the question of death. It began for us in the days after the cancer had metastasized, after the terminal diagnosis which sent us back to the wild-flower meadows of our childhood. I had been messaging her about some things we'd been talking about to reassure one another: the power of comfrey and mistletoe and how what was happening to my sister was chronic not terminal. One of the things I said was: 'We are going to have so much more fun and good times and laugh a lot.'

And then there was a quote I'd seen somewhere, though I wasn't sure where: 'None of us are getting out of here alive.'

Later, when I looked it up, I found that it was attributed to many people including Christopher Walken and also Keanu Reeves, although I somehow doubted it was from him. I think it's by a writer called Nanea Hoffman and my sister liked it. This phrase was good: it was a leveller. My sister was going to die, but so was I. None of us would leave this place alive. I know that idea reassured her, so we'd message it to one another, or say it sometimes in a grim and funny way, to remind us that we were all going towards the same place, it was just that none of us knew the speed of travel there.

I wish I had talked to her a lot more about death. In fact, I wish I had talked to her even once more about death, but she didn't want to discuss it. She said, sometimes, 'I don't like talking about it,' so there was no way I could. You cannot force or coax someone with metastatic cancer to talk to you about what they think of the afterlife. We were both in denial. Perhaps we all are. And how often does death really bring a warning with it? How prepared can you ever be when it arrives? My mum lived on the brink between death and life for twenty-two years after her accident, but that didn't mean I was ready when she died. My sister, we told ourselves, would be the one who would defy all the odds (terrible odds. She had terrible, terrible odds from the moment she was first diagnosed but we absolutely never said this to one another). However predictable, however inevitable, her death was still a complete shock.

A total shock. Even when we went for those appointments in grey hospitals, waiting outside, giggling, experiencing what we both knew was a type of latent hysteria. Even when we walked out of those hospital appointments, when it felt as if trapdoors had suddenly been flung open because the oncologist had tipped his head slightly and said, 'There are still options . . .' his voice trailing off because what could he say? That after the last option, two steps from there, a matter of months, the next option was death?

There was a moment, walking out of the hospital, after my sister was told that she now had secondary cancer, when she had to press her palm to her forehead as we stood beside the car. She was in her long fur coat, and she stood holding the car-door handle in the rain. We had not said anything aloud to one another but quivering in the air between us like a bubble was the thought that this moment was the worst moment. I had felt as if I was in a destroyed world, a terrible world, but now I realize that actually it was a great moment, for we were there, still together. Death hadn't actually come between us yet; I wish I had known then that that moment was actually one of the best. I wish I had known then that the day I was living inside with my sister after her terminal diagnosis was actually everything that life was and all and everything I wanted now. She was still there, inside that day. A day is a good long time when you don't have any of them left.

After she had finished pressing her palm to her face, she said she was fine to drive and that actually she would like to drive, she *wanted* to drive. The first place she drove was to a jeweller where she bought a heavy gold signet ring that cost over a thousand pounds; she was going to buy me one as well that cost four hundred pounds but I said to her not to spend her money although I regret that now. I would love to be wearing a ring my sister had bought me. Then we drove away from Cheltenham and out on to the old Cirencester road, ignoring the bypass from Swindon to Gloucester. Perhaps thundering down a fast bypass seemed something too perilous to undertake at that moment, although we didn't articulate this to one another, we just silently followed the old road, the single carriageway with verges which was the route our school bus used to take.

The gold ring shone dully on my sister's little finger as she held the wheel, and the purple flash of a bank of cyclamen we passed almost took my breath away. We travelled through that afternoon silently and perhaps without think-ing and we arrived at the place where time and memory joined together: the wet, muddy familiar lanes around

Minety, the village where we grew up. There was a rusting dark orange gate in the gap between two hedges where we parked, a silver glint of water from a little gravel stream below us and we did not worry about the wet grass soaking our shoes, but walked into a field where we had played together as children. I have been there many times since I was a child, and each time I go as an adult I am absolutely aware that it is a sort of pilgrimage into the past. To visit is to venture into a kind of acute dome of memory which can be terrifying but is an infinitely beautiful place too. We walked amongst the grass and put our hands into the wet hedges and we talked about Mum and the different ways that we missed her and the ways in which what had happened after her accident had shaped us. But we didn't talk about death and we didn't overtly talk about how we could communicate with one another if one went on ahead before the other. Instead, we talked about the relief of being back in Minety. We talked about how much those wet green fields, with the thick hedges woven with blackthorn and a scattering of wild flowers in the longer grass that grew beneath the hedges, meant to us. We lifted our faces to the cold spring sun whose light hit the ground exactly in the places it had when we were children, and we spread our coats out over the wet ground and ran our hands over the short grass, feeling the earth, breathing, if you like, *with* the ancient, forever earth. We had lost a lot in our lives together but in those moments, in those fields, the past and present were both there. The loss hadn't lessened us but had actually become us.

I am not absolutely sure I even know what my sister

thought about death and whether she believed in another horizon. I know she once said she thought it would be as Einstein had said, that you have no consciousness before you are born and that was OK, and you won't know about it after you've gone, and I mean, yes, I get that, but I've also always felt this was a little bit of a cop-out.

What do you believe in? We should have asked this of one another. Because that question is not really about 'what' but *where*. What we really should have asked each other is, *Do you believe that we will see each other again after we have died? Do you believe we will be present to one another again or is this moment all of it?* Perhaps if I go and walk in that wet field right now and I put my hands into the hedges, watching out for the blackthorn, I might be able to remember everything she said. And if I cannot remember I might be able to feel it because when I am at my most optimistic, I am sure all the messages are waiting there anyway. I wish we had talked about this more clearly and perhaps made notes on it to refer back to later. I'd like to be able to go back to exact notes, written on my phone or in a notepad, of a conversation between us, ideally while we were sitting in that field. Now I don't truly know what she believed. But I believe we will be together again in another place.

After I wrote this for you, I dreamed of my sister again. I was going for communion in a church and she was walking back down the aisle. She didn't really look at me, but I know she knew I was there and her presence was a relief.

Afterwards, when I woke up and was fully dressed, I had to call my father to hear his voice. I loved talking to him. I loved hearing his voice. In the beginning it had been Mum and my dad and my sister and me. Now we were the two who were left.

We talked for an hour. The virus was getting closer and the death it represented was no longer something we could all ignore. We talked about the news that there was going to be a shortage of ventilators and that a company that made cars in Wales was going to start making them. I told him I was very scared by the pictures of people struggling to breathe in hospital wards. We discussed the massive makeshift hospitals going up in London and elsewhere – and the name Nightingale, presumably to reassure but which was actually so chilling – and how this felt as if we were sitting in the path of an approaching apocalypse.

'I don't understand how something so extreme can be happening and yet it feels normal,' I said to my father. Then my father told me he'd lost a notebook.

'A plain black notebook. I left it on the edge of the kitchen table and it's completely vanished. I had it, and now it's gone.' He told me he thought my sister had taken it. 'I think she's close at the moment,' he said, and I loved that thought.

As the virus moved towards us all, unstoppable, and now absolutely visible in the moving images that were appearing on our screens, of wards and wards of patients dying in northern Italy, I was aware of the world moving faster.

There were daily news briefings as the familiar pillars of life fell: offices closed, shops closed, borders closed, schools closed, GCSEs cancelled. After that fast movement there was then complete stillness. A kind of unreality settled as if there had been a massive bomb that had blown the world up and now everyone was in a new landscape in which we sat at home, watching and waiting, as a new reality fell like the red-grey sparks thrown up very fast by a bonfire, which after the fire must settle.

We were all shut in, painfully alone or painfully busy, children tangled maddeningly around feet, some people frantically pummelling homemade bread as if the answer to all this lay in the puffs of the yeasty dough. Put your hands into the earth, people told each other. Those with gardens had it easier than those without, and many people felt that some kind of metaphysical answer to our great shared existential crisis must lie in the soil, although this wasn't a feeling I shared.

And death, and the journey around it, seemed to have become everyone's business, quite suddenly. It was unsettling that the roulette wheel was now spinning in front of everyone and the die was jumping around. None of us knew where it would settle, and everyone was scared. People posted stories on their social media channels about grief, and how we were all grieving. I felt a bit affronted, as if a lot of people had suddenly moved into a front room I'd been quietly sitting in on my own, or with a few other, very special people. Now I had to share sofas, floor space and the air I was breathing. I didn't feel all these people necessarily deserved this space. I had been trying to work out what death really was – my own little project – and suddenly all these other people were too. A friend who lives in a house on the edge of a village in Wiltshire, and who is married with children and all her closest family still alive, texted me that lockdown was the hardest thing she had ever experienced. I stared at her text and thought of her living sisters and brother and mother and father and decided she definitely didn't deserve any floor space in my room.

But there were people who really needed the space: someone who I had worked with whose teenage daughter died at the bottom of an empty concrete swimming pool nine months ago, or another whose newly married son has just been diagnosed with MS, or the friend whose sister is dying of a brain tumour. They needed it. Even so, I felt crowded.

By the end of March everything was extraordinary and also completely boring. Suddenly people were actually using their phones to make and receive phone calls and speak to each other, talking incessantly about how weird life was and that it was like the war and also that they could feel the earth breathing a sigh, although it wasn't clear to me if that sigh was of relief or irritation.

Partly to assuage my own irritation and partly in response to the sudden closure of schools, I decided to rearrange the shelves in the kitchen so that any books we had that vaguely related to home-schooling were all in one place. Evangeline found herself a small table from amongst the junk in an upstairs cupboard. She set this up in the kitchen, with her own pot of pens and files. On the bookshelves I swapped unread novels for *A Children's Guide to History*, *A First Book of Wild Flowers*, a world atlas, *What the Pagans Do*, and *My Book of Practical Science*. It was satisfying when Pete wrote up a timetable on the chalk-board in the kitchen even though we all then ignored it. There was so much for us all to do in this completely new world where very little happened.

It was so, so weird. Everything was so weird. Of course, we talked about this with all of the children, but we had been through so much already, they knew what death was, they knew what death takes away. They knew what death had done to us and how it had made them feel. I did not, therefore, dwell with them on the idea that more of the people we love so much could be in danger. I thought of my father and stepmother and put them in my mind into a place of safety. The world had stopped and when I lay on the grass outside the kitchen, since it was strangely, unseasonably warm for spring, the blue sky was just bright, bright blue. There were no criss-cross marks of planes ploughing through it. There was no traffic on the road by our house and there were no trains running down the track at the end of our garden.

My teenagers walked through the house looking a little like I felt much of the time now: lost and stunned, a whole future they'd been visualizing just shearing away like a rock from a hillside.

They did not talk about death. They talked about life. They wanted to see their friends. They wanted life to resume.

'When will things get back to normal? How long do you think it will take?' Dolly asked, kneeling down on the grass beside me, pushing her hair, a long curtain, back over her shoulders.

Ah, that's the question, Dolly! How long will it take? When will we go back to normal?

Where was the portal backwards? Everyone was looking for it. Everyone wanted the car that had stalled and seemed broken to splutter back into life and the world to start revolving again and the planes to start flying and the people to walk in and out of the heated shops to buy hair serum in plastic tubes and speakers encased in plastic wrapping and a very expensive handbag that was never really needed.

I lay on the grass beside Dolly, who was kneeling up, cutting across the sun, and closed my eyes to the blue, blue sky. We were all knights, now, and we had ventured into the darkest part of the forest and there was no route back from here. Time travel hadn't yet been invented and neither had resurrection. None of us could go back. Only onwards. Only forward. I pressed my body into the spring earth and imagined for a moment I could feel the world revolving.

However dark the forest was, this was what I had now learned. We cannot go backwards. We go forwards, out-wards. We are not merely bystanders to death but creating our own relationship with it. The object of understanding death is not to look backwards but to understand who you are in relation to the world without the dead person in it. The truth is that the death and therefore loss of someone you love deeply is so awful you have to rearrange your brain dramatically to survive it. You are thrown into pieces that you have to reconfigure in order to go on living. But that reconfiguration also might be metaphysical (like all the poetry that kept arriving for me) or supernatural (like the ghost I was trying and failing to call up). Whether I would ever reach or meet the metaphysical or supernatural was still not clear, but I was gaining a sense that the death of my sister could possibly force me to create a life that was other than the one that I had had before. And perhaps that life would be brighter; perhaps I would be able to create a force field around my existence that would mean my life might become stronger, bolder, more colourful and much more perilous but also vivid. And that would be *because of* having been in the room with death, not *despite* having been in the room with death.

I thought about plunging into the winter-cold river water and how it had challenged the state of homeostasis – that is, the optimum and steady state – in which my body had started the day. Cold water had shocked me but when I emerged from it I'd felt more alive, even if the fact of feeling more alive was the fact of feeling more pain. Because I was also learning that the more pain I felt, the more poetry I felt, too. Sometimes I think that an easy life might be worse than death. A homeostatic life might *feel* like death. I did not want a steady life. And I had begun to feel that the only way to affirm life was to affirm the darkness of it at exactly the same time as I felt its bright warmth. I said these things to Dolly and I told her that if we wanted to find a way to exist that we liked, we would have to create a new place, not return to the old world. She frowned, watching me as I lay on my back, one hand shielding my eyes from the sharp sun. From an upstairs bedroom I could hear Dash shouting something about Lego. Dolly flicked her eyes up to the window, then back to me.

'We have to change. We have to find, I don't know exactly, but something new, a new way of living,' I told her, and I wasn't sure if I was referring to Covid and the new life it had brought with it, or simply death. 'Just because we're faced with a challenge doesn't mean we'll rise to it. There's no guarantee that what we're going through now will make us stronger, better. But if we know that, at least there's more chance we can evolve from it, and not just go back. We can't go back to normal.'

Dolly brushed away a strand of hair that was sticking to the shiny salve of her lips. Then she stood up, brushing dried grass from her legs.

'I think it's exciting. I mean, it's terrible. Obviously the virus is terrible, but learning to live in a new way. I don't want to go backwards either, Mum. I want to go forward, with you. And anyway. We have to make lunch now.'

The shouting continued from an upstairs bedroom, but there was a sudden gust of wind too so that inside a door slammed. Still lying on the grass, pressed into the earth, I shut my eyes, but through the lids I could feel the outline of the sun above me. I needed to make time move forward, just as I had told Dolly.

It was still warm and light in the evening, and after supper I wandered around the garden, picking up clothes the

children had left behind – draped over the backs of chairs
or in a rumple beside the paddling pool, where they'd
stepped straight out of them. I gathered up the clothes and
then gathered up the children, pulling T-shirts over their
curls, buttoning them reluctantly back into their shorts.

I wanted to walk out of the house with them, to escape
a feeling of time as a circular track within. Despite the sunshine outside, lockdown had a habit of making us all pace
around our homes like caged dogs, searching for bones to
gnaw at for meaning. I had to stop pacing and walk, somewhere, even if this had to be at the pace of the children.
Which is, slow.

'Come on,' I said, 'we are going out to find magic.'

They mewed and complained back at me, Dash and
Lester rushing away to fill their hands with Lego men. They
all knew my search for magic, when said in that certain
voice, actually just meant walking down the green by the
house, to the medieval church. They didn't see this as
magic, just a slightly boring walk they did all the time.

None of them were wearing socks, but Dash and Evangeline ran ahead as I held Lester's hand and he complained
bitterly about how bored he was, how hungry he was, how
he needed a small glass of water. I had made fishcakes for
supper, but Lester had not wanted any of them. Instead, I
gave him bites from an apple I'd picked up as we left the
kitchen, as we walked along the narrow concrete path that
ran down the green by our house.

Evangeline and Dash were peering at us over the top of
a gravestone when Lester and I got to the churchyard.

Evangeline was two when we moved to the village, Dash was a baby and Lester was born two years later. We have to walk through the churchyard to get to the field down the green which we rent to keep our ponies in, so they have grown up walking backwards and forwards through the churchyard many times a week. It's a place where they play, or hunt for conkers, and sometimes if there's been a storm we take handfuls of sticks that have fallen on to the grass to light the red stove in the pink playroom at home. In this way my children are acquainted with the symbols of death, and it's how I grew up, too, as my childhood home was next door to the church in our village. A tall wall was all that separated the garden where we played from the graves. The first time I sat on the edge of my bed as a child and touched myself until I came, I was staring out of the window at gravestones.

So I wasn't surprised that Dash and Evangeline had already started playing hide-and-seek behind the graves when I arrived with Lester, who was still complaining bitterly about boredom. A gravestone is the perfect size for a medium-sized child to curl up behind. Harder for an adult, but there were tall, straight horse chestnut trees in the graveyard I could hide behind, and often the children didn't think of looking behind them when it was my turn.

The evening was soft, still, and the children's voices, rising and falling in the dusk as they chased each other, were the only sound.

Lester could not keep up with Dash and Evangeline so I took him to the church door, turning the huge round metal handle, and really expecting it to be locked, since the virus had meant everything was locked, shut out, shut down, but it gave in my hand. I pushed the door with my palm and noticed properly for the first time the big metal nails driven through it, which might have been there for several hundred years. Light from the clear glass windows spilled on to the cool stone floor but the church was completely still.

I felt Lester's small hand tighten in mine as we walked inside, where silence hung in the air, the moment suspended. Lester made a sound, testing the silence, and his voice echoed so he did it again. I let the curtain over the door fall back, so for that moment we were cocooned within the walls of the church, the rise and fall of Dash and Evangeline's voices shut out. We walked up the nave, touching pews, the stone walls, because there was something reassuring in the ancient presence of the medieval building around us. On one window there was a pot of white chrysanthemums placed where the sunlight spilled in; it was surrounded by small petals and three dead flies, but it was life still. Outside I heard the children's voices, increasingly loud, as they called for me, and I picked Lester up on to my hip, telling him, 'Come on, let's find them.' On the wall opposite the door was the faded outline of a mural. I pointed to it, showing Lester, without saying anything, the outline of a man on a horse, his long sword thrown back behind him, and a woman standing before him. It was a faded burgundy colour but six hundred years ago it had been a painting of a knight.

When we came out, the children were waiting for us. I

started counting, so that they knew it was my turn to seek them, their voices shrieking and then falling as they ran further away from me, around the far side of the church. I ran after them, in imitation of seeking, as I knew exactly where they were. However old I become, I will always associate this churchyard with the green smell of the box hedge in the drive of the house beside it. Running now through the churchyard, feigning frustration that I couldn't find them, then pouncing on them so that they shrieked and laughed and laughed so much that their voices echoed around, rising and falling in the last light of the day, I felt happy, as if all the dark rooks had flown away.

When we had finished playing we stopped for a moment and the children were suddenly standing very still beside the glossy green leaves of the laurel bush near the church door. Dash said he missed my sister, and when I looked at Evangeline I could see tears were glinting on her face. She put her hand out, brushing the edge of the green leaves, then snatching her hand back because there was a sound like rustling inside the leaves, as if they had been moved, not by the wind, but by something inside them. Evangeline said, 'What do you think that was?' And then she said, '*Who* do you think that was?' Because it was not just me that had seen it. I smiled at her. Lester tugged on my hand as Dash had run away, leaving the wooden gate swinging open.

There was a moon in the sky as we walked back to the house, and the barn owl with the round human face swooped back over the dark field. I saw I had a choice. I could try to turn that thing that sometimes made me feel as if I might pass out with pain – that is, my sister's death – into the thing that might make me want to live more of this life. I could turn away, or I could choose to see, and even go out to look for, more ancient outlines of knights, and glossy green leaves, and owls with human and beautiful faces.

Later that night I had been asleep for some hours when I woke up suddenly with a sense my sister was tapping on my shoulder. I sat up very quickly, feeling sweat underneath my breasts. She had been there, and she was not there, and I sat in bed worrying very deeply about how her body might be now, over three months after she had been buried. I wanted to wake Pete up and ask him if he thought that she might start manifesting herself to me more strongly at the same time as her physical body was disintegrating, or perhaps had already gone. I didn't know how long it took for a human body to break down. When I turned around in bed Pete wasn't there, but I could hear the sound of a screen, the rolling blur of news, from the kitchen downstairs. I felt steady when I put my bare feet on to my bedroom floor, but in the bathroom there was an outline of shadow cast into the bright white of the bath from a geranium plant I had taken from her house. I didn't switch the bathroom light on as there was a whiteness from the full moon. I drank straight from the tap, leaning forward so that my eye line was level with the bathroom shelves. When I had been in my sister's house, I had taken some things from her bathroom which otherwise would have gone into the bin – some little bottles of essential oil, some chestnut shampoo, a face oil. Also on the shelf in my bathroom was a tube of a gel called bioXtra Dry Mouth, which the nurses in the hospital had given us as she lay dying and which I had wiped on to her tongue in those last hours. I didn't know what to do with it. When I stood up and wiped my mouth, I looked at the tube, which said 'Comforts and Protects'. Perhaps if I kept it, I might stay closer to my sister. I had worried that if I threw it carelessly in the bin, it might suggest a lack of care for her. I wasn't sure. In the darkness I turned to go back to bed. As I did, I noticed there were no crimson petals growing on the geranium now, just the shadow cast into the bottom of the white bath of the bent outline of its stalk, in the shape of a human bone.

Chapter 5

Just a Star

In my search for my sister and also for the person I should become now that she, and also the people we had been in relation to one another, were gone, it was tempting to look for clues in all the messages, emails, notifications my sister and I had sent each other. I was looking for hidden meaning in all our many, many forms of communication. I also looked around for bits of her handwriting. In the cupboard in my bedroom there was a card she'd written to me just after the opening night of her last circus show. The card said:

Darling Clover and Pete Thank you for all your help, support and enthusiasm with opening night. To good times this summer lets hope the sun is still like this by the time we all end up on the river at Lechlade together – I am looking forward to that! LOVE LOVE

Her writing was optimistic and in some ways easier to look at than the digital typed messages. The cards were final, they did not invite an immediate reply, unlike the digital messages which left the sense of a flashing cursor, a possibility I found too sad to think of. The messages on my phone were more likely to play tricks on me too. One day I was on WhatsApp and a notification popped up saying 'Tap to chat' with my sister's name beside it. I threw the phone down on to the bed, shocked that my phone seemed to think my sister might still be alive. At another time I looked at a group we had both been part of and a message popped up telling me she had left the group. Again this shocked me. I had her phone in my cupboard. I knew that no one else had it, so I did not understand how she had been able to leave the group. Yet another time, I found myself distractedly blowing a kiss to one of the last emojis she had ever sent me. There was a message between us on Facebook that I had not replied to and I hated seeing that message. She had sent me a funny image of a face-distortion app with herself wearing a pirate's hat and she wanted me to see it. She had written:

Hey clo
Bit weird but look at this selfi thingy
Super super bored in nial bar
But it makes me look like you?!?
No need to reply to this very important message! XXXX

Maybe I had not seen it. Maybe I had been busy or distracted but I had not answered.

*

One thing I found myself doing more often than reading her messages was trying to talk aloud to my sister. I use the word 'found' since it wasn't really something I set out to do. I didn't set out to go on a walk to try to shift the sadness I felt and talk to her as I walked. I didn't purposefully talk to her as I led one of the ponies back down to its paddock. I didn't mean to say her name and ask her where she was as I put clothes away in the drawers. It was something I found myself doing. I will admit that often this made me feel extremely embarrassed; even, weirdly, ashamed. Shame is not a familiar sensation for me, so I am not quite sure where this feeling came from, except an uncomfortable sense I was trying to test my sister. She was dead and I shouldn't be trying to test her: that should be saved for life, shouldn't it? You can't test someone in death. Or perhaps I was trying to test God, or the universe or fate or destiny.

Whoever I was addressing, I was definitely trying to perform some kind of cosmic or soul test. Sometimes I thought that if I spoke to her loudly enough, or firmly enough, or just enough enough, our shared past would appear before me like a shimmering hologram. I wanted to believe that when I spoke to her I would actually be able to feel her, if not see her, and with her feel all the life we'd lived through together. Remember, I'd been so worried about losing that life I'd wanted to lock it into a silver chest. But of course, however much I talked away, there was never going to be a hologram, and so while I was certainly trying to test something – maybe myself in fact – I kept finding life around me wanting. The test was endlessly failed. What I wanted and could never find, kept failing to find, was any certainty. A loud and clear and positive answer.

Often I thought of the fact that I wished I had talked to my sister about how she might embody herself when she was dead. Again, this is not a conversation I ever had with her; it was too late to have it with her, anyway, by the time her cancer had metastasized. But it would be a useful conversation to have with people you love. I think it's one that I need to have with my children soon. Wouldn't it be nice to say, 'I will return to you in the form of *this thing*. So when you see *this thing* you can be sure that it's me.'

When I chat with people on Instagram about their experience of death, we often talk about how seeing this butterfly or that robin is immensely comforting. We want to believe. We want certainty that the lost dead person is present in our ongoing lives. But, as a result, it seems to me that we invest robins and butterflies with an almost solemn and hugely overloaded responsibility to be the people we love. There are a LOT of people flying around in robins. I wonder, is this just because robins are pretty and we like to think of them as sort of sociable? Although I am not sure how sociable they really are. When I started my pathetic attempt to grow vegetables during lockdown, I noticed many robins, but they were not actually being friendly. They were simply wanting to come to the area where the soil had been turned over and was freshest and wettest, as that's where the worms would be. They were coming to eat – that is, kill – worms. When you think about it like this, it's funny really, isn't it, that we all want to embody our missing sister and nan and dad in these little killer birds. And I wonder, often, why we do not embody the people we love in other kinds of creatures. Is it only because the robin and butterfly are pretty? Why does no one recognize their loved one in a calf or a dog or a pigeon, for example? There are a lot of those around so rationally it should be more comforting than seeking out a vicious little robin looking for worms. I mean, if I felt I could see my sister in a pigeon, I could just go to Trafalgar Square and she would be EVERY-WHERE and rather overbearing. Actually, sometimes I think she is a storm, when it whips up and is everywhere, raging, as if she's trying to reassert herself into my life.

More often, however, when I tried to talk to her I felt I was clutching at an idea that didn't even exist. It made me feel stupid.

One evening I was sitting outside my house in the dark, smoking a cigarette. The night was very dark and there were no twinkling stars or storm to talk to. There was noth-ing to focus my mind and nowhere to look for her, let alone find her. But I was searching, wondering, and the alarm that had been in my head so much – whereareyou whereareyou whereareyou – was going off so I tried talking to her. It was one of those moments when I felt a bit embarrassed, almost as if I could see myself from a distance and I looked ridicu-lous, talking into the dark. But maybe that's the thing about death: when we get close to it, it does make us look ridicu-lous by stripping away everything we are and leaving us in our most human, most vulnerable state. And because we are at our most vulnerable, the fact of looking what might be considered ridiculous under normal circumstances – tear-stained, with puffy and squinty eyes and flailing, like a fish gasping for breath on the riverbank – doesn't matter. We show everything of ourselves when we are close to death and so at that moment we are also most human. Most human and therefore most wonderful and magnificent.

What I didn't realize then, though, was that the thing I thought was embarrassing about me at that moment was also what was most beautiful about me, and that thing was the grace of my humanity that existed alongside my disbelief, rage, hurt. I just felt alone and ridiculous, even though I was still open to talking to my sister. And I called her name and tried to just talk to her. I wasn't at all comfortable. I heard my own voice, which was much too loud, but nothing from her. I felt no sense of her. And then I sort of felt like saying to myself, *What do you expect? What do you expect, you stupid human person? Do you honestly expect the dense black to start glowing, or a star to start winking at you? Are you looking for that kind of certainty?*

Instead, I just shivered, and the night felt dark and damp, but just then there was a gust of wind. And noise: a piece of dried-up holly that I had put behind a picture at Christmas and then thrown outside the kitchen door with the Christmas tree that Jimmy had burnt, but which had remained lying on the wooden boards outside the kitchen door, was lifted and moved across the wood. And at that moment, I gasped, for there it was, there was my sign, there was my certainty, because when I looked up at the velvet darkness, one bright, bright golden star had appeared in the black night.

And then I stubbed my cigarette out and I thought: Often, what terrifies me most is not that I'm wrong, but that I am right. And if I am right, it means I am seeing you in all these signs. And can that really be true?

Is that the truth I have been looking for?

That you in all your blazing glory are now simply a star.

A star?

That's all?

Later I realized why speaking her name and trying to make her answer made me feel sort of ashamed and scared, and that was because it was as if I was chasing her. In talking to her I was trying to follow her. It reminded me of the times when we were children and we played hide-and-seek. We grew up in a house that might have been designed for games like this. It was like the kind of house my children construct out of old boxes when we do that thing children call 'junk modelling'. (Actually, it's just sticking pieces of rubbish together, but Evangeline, Dash and Lester love doing it.) Our house was a bit like that: big, but not grand, and there were two staircases and lots of hidden cupboards and tiny rooms that opened off the backs of one another through endless doors. There was an outside room up some stone steps separate from the house that Mum called the apple room, as it was where she stored all the apples that had fallen from the trees around the house for the winter.

So it was a great house for a child to grow up and play in,

as we could evade the adults easily, escape into our own worlds, and also create dens and camps in those worlds, which would not be found and tidied away for ages. It was a warren, and this warren was the place where I played with my sister. But sometimes she'd hide so effectively, in the apple room or the cupboard under the stairs – where we'd once found a nest of dead mice and which had scared me ever since, but not her – that I'd lose her. And I'd walk through the house calling her name. Calling for her, looking for her, until I'd realize that I'd looked everywhere, and what I had to do was abandon the hunt and turn around and leave her.

When I sat outside my house and talked at her into the night and heard nothing, or when I rode my horse through the fields by the house and shouted her name into the wind, it reminded me of the same feeling. She had evaded me. She had deserted me. She was gone, just as she had, sometimes, when she hid from me as a child and I was left to wander back through the house, to return to the kitchen, to leave our game and the world we were inhabiting alone together, and turn back into my own world. Her death was giving me the same feeling of defeated disappointment. But I started to realize that part of the work I had to do was to stop calling her name and to leave her where she was hidden from me, at least for the moment. I knew I'd come back and hunt for her, reach for her again, but now it was time to turn around and go back into my own life. To go and have supper with the children and Pete. To go and look after and love the living.

*

Navigating through that spring was helped by the fact that the weather was epic, which created a feeling of change even though none of us could go anywhere. We were not really supposed to leave our houses. Perhaps it was the most beautiful spring that had ever happened. Certainly it felt like it. Everything else was really weird and very bad – my sister had died, there was a virus flying around the world which meant that touching anything or even breathing in had become dangerous, and everyone was shut in – but day after day dawn rolled around like a surreal technicolour dream of yellow and orange. Some days, if I couldn't sleep, I'd get up and drive to the Ridgeway, walking alone along the slice of white chalk path on the top of the bright green hills. The landscape had changed and was no longer hard and dark but now unnaturally rich, frothy with may and cow parsley as skylarks burst the silence with their wings and movement. But the human landscape below the moving sky was still. There were no cars on the M4 and no trains on the tracks that I could see from the furthest top of the hills.

Up on the hill I increasingly resisted the urge to talk to my sister. That weird embarrassment I felt was there quite often and, anyway, I was thinking of her so much that NOT talking to her was a relief. Maybe it was this new stillness that had come over us all because of the virus, as we lost that mad urge to dash around, but a few weeks into lockdown my sister was suddenly, unexpectedly, absolutely everywhere. When I shut my eyes at night it felt as if she swept into my brain and was sitting there, quietly, watching me and not saying anything. In my brain I saw flashes of her, but more than anything I felt her presence in my head, all the time. When I woke up, before I opened my eyes it was as if she was tapping on the inside of my eyelids, willing me to wake up. My mum used to tell us a story about the moment my sister first came to see me in hospital when I was a baby. I was wrapped up in a waffle blanket in one of those clear plastic cribs beside our mum's bed, and my sister tapped on the side of the cot and said, 'Wake up, Clover, wake up and look at my new jersey.' It felt as if something a bit like that was happening now, only the tapping she was doing was not on a plastic box after my birth, but on the inside of my eyelids after her death.

The weird part about this was that I didn't want her to be there. I spent a lot of my days thinking of her and wanting her but now I didn't want her suddenly inside my brain or pressing at my eyes. When she started tapping, every morning before I was properly awake, I felt really tired. I wanted the reality of her death to go away. I didn't want her behind my eyelids. I didn't want her blackly on the inside of my brain. She had become my fixation since I thought about her the whole time, and that felt as if I had no time when I wasn't thinking about her. She was the ticker tape whirling about in my brain that wouldn't rest. I didn't want to think of her or be with her like this. I wanted to open my eyes when I woke up (with no tippy-tap from her inside my eyelids) and for it to just be a normal day, without a dead sister and her death to wrestle with.

I still often, during the day, reached for my phone to text her about something, before that horrible, hard, falling feeling of the remembering hit me. Sometimes, I still sent her photographs. After I had persuaded Jimmy to come riding with me, I sent my sister a picture of us together, on our horses, because I knew she would want to see that.

'You never know,' I said to Pete.

More than anything, I wanted to just be able to call her on the phone and maybe chat for a bit or even have a full-blown argument, as we often did. A call might end with one of us hanging up on the other, or just going silent. Look, we were – we are – sisters. We fought. We loved each other. That was how our relationship worked. There were all the emotions, and all the intimacy that's needed to be everything to one another. It was constant communication, even when we were not talking. And there were fights – huge blow-ups that made my heart pound and left my shoulders heaving with sobs – but a day later we'd be texting about a plan to be together, just as if this was normal. Because it was normal.

Now that her memories were everywhere, my home, my refuge, became uncomfortable. When I woke up, I had to battle against them pressing on me. The house was full of places I remembered her. The last time she had ever been there, sitting in the kitchen with Dash on her lap as she brushed his hair, as white-blond as her own. The wall of pictures she'd hung in the sitting room, leaving a little beaded Indian bag over one of them I was always afraid someone would move, since it was so important to me that the last hands to have touched it had been hers. The place where her car pulled up into the drive and she leant from the window and kissed me on the lips; the window she pointed out of, from the kitchen, and said, 'There, plant a rose there.' Now, though, these memories were not pleasant. They pinched and hurt me, like soft skin suddenly caught in a zip.

And every morning I'd awake with a sense of *here we go again*. Here we go again into the dizzying, exhausting, unceasing thoughts of her and wondering where she was. She was always there, in my head, and absolutely nowhere to be found.

Being locked in with these big feelings was difficult. There was no minotaur waiting for me behind a door any more. The physiological isolation I had felt so intensely in the first days after she had died, as if I alone had taken acid, had gone. And that sense of a mild poisoning, in the further weeks after her death, was passing too. I could walk around the house in a normal way now. I wasn't hunched. I could put mascara on and know that sometimes, at the end of the day, it'd still be there. I could answer the door to a DHL delivery driver and not have to tell him (rarely a her) that my sister had recently died, which was why my signature was illegible. In some ways, not having to commune with the rest of the world, such as at the school gate or even at the supermarket, since going shopping now was a major deal that only happened every couple of weeks rather than every few days, was a big relief. There were no parties. I think this mostly was a good thing. For someone who has recently been up close with death, going to a party is a really strange thing. I went to a Christmas party three weeks after my mother had died in 2013 and it felt as if everyone's faces had become slightly exaggerated versions of themselves: lips redder, hair blacker and so on, and the noise in the room was as if it had been turned up inside my ear. I was relieved, really, that there were absolutely no parties that springtime, and yet having no place to go was also confusing. It might have been nice, occasionally, to dilute my feelings amongst a big crowd, but that wasn't a possibility. Sometimes, too, I worried that I might have completely lost my ability to even be with other people at all.

But still, I knew that being at home, moving between the garden and the kitchen ceaselessly for weeks, wasn't allowing me to be witness to the way I felt about my sister's death in the same way I would have conceived it if I was out in the world. I wanted a task to take my feelings to. It was my birthday during lockdown, a sunny day when I went riding with Dash, and Jimmy made supper, and Evangeline played cards with me and Pete gave me a gold disc with all the children's names engraved on it so I would always have the names of those five people I loved most in the world close to me. I felt as if I might be happy, but I wasn't sure if I was enacting the way someone ought to be feeling, rather than actually feeling something. I was also afraid of taking myself to a place away from my sister. I was afraid of the feeling that I could actually be happy. And I realized that what I was also trying to find, in learning to be happy again, was the new path I'd walk which ran between the relationship I had had with her when she was alive – all forty-four years of that time – and the new path I was being forced to walk, now she was dead.

When I wrote that last sentence I first wrote forty-five. That is because forty-five is the age I am at *this* moment in time. But forty-four is the age I was when my sister died in December 2019. I wish I had been forty-five and not forty-four. I wish I had been fifty-five or sixty-five or – best – eighty-five. I am not completely 100 per cent sure either of us really wanted to live to ninety-five, but who knows. Fifty-five would have been so much better than forty-five. If I had been fifty-five and she had been fifty-seven then we would truly have been adults together. If we'd got to fifty-five and fifty-seven together alive, and then leant forward much further, we'd have been at sixty. As it is, I feel as if I can stretch backwards and we as adolescents are still there; the very tips of my fingers can just brush us. When I look back at that little glimpse of life that came before death, I feel as if we were only just getting going. We'd done a lot – building lives and making work, several marriages and seven children – but I still feel as if we were only just skating into adult life. And also, all that working, birthing, marrying, divorcing, loving, etc. had made us so busy. I wish we'd had more time to be adults together. I wish we had had the long coast beyond fifty. When I look forward, from this point, at forty-five, I always imagine it might get a little bit easier after fifty. No very small children needing wiping, lifting, feeding, and hopefully some sense of having reached a point of knowing what we were good at. I wish we had been in our fifties together. It'd be too much to ask the universe to be old people together. I cannot imagine myself in old age, and since my mother, two aunts and sister were all dead before they got there, I don't truthfully imagine it's a place I'll be alive in either. So I do not beg the universe to give me the years we would have had together as old people, for they are inconceivable, but I would so much like to have been in the middle of life with my sister. I didn't know my mother as an adult. I never had an adult conversation with her. And now I realize I will never have another adult conversation with either of these two most important women in my life.

As a way of trying to communicate, by putting my hands into the past, I went back to the place that would cause me the most pain. I willingly took myself into the vortex, to Minety, the damp, low-lying village where we grew up. Like Gawain I knew I had a challenge I must rise to. There is a wood there called Flisteridge, which to me is like a stage or the place of a dream perhaps. It's hard just to call up magical thinking but when I want to, I go to Minety, or to Flisteridge, or the wild-flower field my sister and I needed to go to on the day we heard that death had moved closer to her. I thought that this would be a good place to start trying to work out who she was and who I was and who WE were together now that one of us was alive and one of us was dead. I had to take the children with me as it was a Sunday, and Pete was shut in, working.

Driving through southern England still gave me the strange sense that an everyday apocalypse had recently been under way, since there was little traffic, no cyclists in bright Dayglo colours to pass, no cafe to stop at near Swindon to buy a cup of coffee. We had been at home for so long, with so few trips anywhere (apart from my occasional journeys to Tesco alone, while Dolly looked after the children at home), that being out in the landscape felt a bit like venturing into a new world. The distances and horizons looked further than they had in the past. The hedges were greener, the cow parsley frothier, the may flowers in the hedges a brighter white. And the children thought we seemed to be moving so fast, since none of them had travelled any faster than walking pace, or maybe at the speed of their little bikes down the green near home. Driving to Minety the first time, I felt as if they joined me on the journey. The path beside death had until then felt pretty solitary.

When we arrived at the woods I parked in the familiar gateway I've been to many times, and we walked, slowly, down the rutted track with pylons running above it, the children complaining it was far, far too long, splashing through silver puddles to the edge of the wood, where the trees went dark green, and the track gave way to another path, snaking through leaf mould, brambles and bracken, where my sister and I had walked and ridden on our ponies many, many times as children. I knew that wood. Memory and a sense of home led me to the violet-blue glow where the bluebells became a continual carpet of colour, covering the green and brown of the leaves, brambles and earth. This was a beautiful place, bucolic England, and Dash and Evangeline ran ahead of me, shouting to one another that they might be the first one to spot Bambi, since the scene was so beautiful, it was like a cartoon. Dolly was with me, Lester clasping her hand, and I could hear her talking to him about colours, and how to spell blue and how to spell bell. Dash and Evangeline kept hunting for Bambi and the smell of the bluebells was so strong, intoxicating almost, as if it were artificial. There was the rope swing, blue nylon tied around a log, where the children played, pushing one another backwards and forwards, and I found the clearing, close to a pheasant feeder, where I stopped, gasping for a moment, because this scene and the smell of the bluebells and their blueness was making me feel dizzy. If I listened closely enough, could I hear the past?

I walked away from the children, off the path, stepping carefully through the bluebells on an undisturbed route, deeper into the wood where oak trees twisted above me, their branches spread out across the big blue sky so that I felt they would catch me when I fell. Because now I was falling, unsure if the ground and the bracken would hold me, the ground beneath my feet uneven, as I tried to find the gap between the trees where my sister and I used to start our races, when we rode here on our ponies. And there was a rushing sound in my head, and I felt my breath all short and cold in my chest, and I could feel something pumping beneath my jersey and I knew it was my heart.

My heart was beating faster and the sound in my head was the rush of red blood through my body, and now the bluebells smelt almost cloyingly sweet – too sweet and sickly. When I tipped back my head the branches and the trees and the sky spun above me, a kaleidoscope of green and brown-blue revolving above my head. When I brought my eyes back down again, it was as if the woodland, the trees, the branches, were all burning, with bright red and orange flames licking upwards, a wall of fire and destruction moving slowly but continually towards me, growing redder and hotter as I faced it. This place deep within the English countryside and deeper within my brain felt like a site of great peril. The memories were so close, so searing, if I'd been wearing no shoes I might have cut my feet on them like shards of broken glass. I felt as if the fire of my memories of being here with my sister would burn me. And what I felt too, which was strange, was that although I was in the furnace, right there inside it so that it burned my face, there was a comfort in it. There was a comfort in feeling so close to death. It was a frightening place to be but in some ways these very close memories enabled me to step over – into, perhaps – the separating place of death. As I walked deeper into the woodland, I knew that I was walking closer to death. Not my own death, of course – I wasn't going to die there – but I was taking myself right up against my sister and in doing so I felt as if I was transcending the separation death had imposed on us. I was allowing the heat to scorch me and it hurt, oh how that heat hurt me, but I was not afraid of it. I was feeling all the pain and I was not afraid of it.

When I shut my eyes, not hard, but very gently, so that I

could feel on my eyeballs the bright glints of afternoon sun as it slashed through the oak branches, I could hear the voices of myself and my sister in the past. Children's voices amongst the sweet, violet intensity of the carpet of flowers that surrounded me, conversing, communicating with each other. I could hear and feel my sister and me as children, chattering, laughing, calling to one another, a rise and fall of voices which I now felt myself leaning into, listening, straining for familiar patterns, words I understood or feelings I could navigate. It was like listening to voices in another room, just out of earshot, or being played backwards, or forwards, but fast forwards, too fast. I could not make out what they were saying. And then the relief that I felt fell away as I realized I still couldn't see, I still couldn't hear, I still couldn't – duh! – reach through the veil, or really grasp where the other place I was looking for lay.

'Can you see meeeee? Muuuuuuum, Mum, Muuuuum, watch meeee,' I could now hear my children shouting. 'Can you seeeee meeeeeeee? Can youuuuuuuuu? Seeeeeeeeeee? Meeeeeeee?'

A small hand tugged my coat, and Evangeline was beside me, hauling me backwards, into her world.

'Did you see me? On the swing? Did you see me going so high? Higher than Dash. Higher than the trees. Mum?'

I blinked harder, wrenching myself back to Evangeline in her yellow anorak and blue trainers and her leggings that had thunderbolts on them with the rip on the knee, back to the present. But I didn't want to have to come back to the present, the moment in time where my children wanted me. I wanted to allow myself to surrender. That is what my friend Liz had said: 'Bow down. Death will always win.'

I had to concentrate on the drive home, stopping to get petrol and take Dash into the garage to use the toilet, and then buy a packet of biscuits for them to share in the car, and it all made me forget about the furnace and the burning wall of pain and the distant voices I might have answered if I could only have heard them properly. I realized that figuring out my relationship with my dead sister and how I could live with her and without her was something I had to do on my own, most of the time. It wasn't helpful for my children if the furnace was too close to them. I don't mean they should not ever see me cry. Crying, I felt – I still feel – is quite healthy, as long as it wasn't all the time. Crying was something we could do together. As long as I wasn't continually splashing salt tears into their tomato soup as I cooked it for them or bursting the bubbles in their baths as tears fell from my face, crying was not a bad thing. Crying has an element of domestication. In a way, I think that when I cried it made the separating pain of death easier for us all to manage within our lives together as there is stuff you can do when another person cries. If I cried, I know it shocked Evangeline a bit but it was also the time she could clamber on to my lap, pressing her face into mine, stroking my hair, as I had done to her so many times. Crying needed cuddles and a cup of tea and maybe some tissues. I cried with Dolly and Evangeline, quite often, simply lying on my bed, after Dash and Lester were asleep. Crying was, in some ways, more contained than the stunned place of far distance that death pulled me into. Crying was anchoring. To see pain, to feel pain, to be present to pain and then to alchemize pain into beautiful life seems to me to be something deeply important for any human being to learn to do in their existence. Maybe it's the most important thing any of us can learn.

But when I was being stalked by death, chasing my sister, being chased by her, woken by her, tapped on my eyelids and sent into the furnace, which were all things that happened in the course of a normal day, I am certain I was a much more difficult woman to have as a mother. And although I knew that death was something they were aware of – how could they not be? – I didn't want to scare them. Instead, I realized I was doing well in my quest through the dark and frightening forest because I was learning how to walk around with death inside me. I was now able to withstand whole days walking around with it there in my chest, like a strange and remarkably terrible fact I thought of all the time but didn't want to share with my children and Pete in case it ruined their day.

Of course there was a fundamental problem with the idea that I could go and experience my grief in a controlled place, away (mostly) from family life, because the waves of grief are not something you can anticipate, like the tides, or schedule in, like a dentist appointment. On some days I could be aware of living through several hours, even half a day, and then a whole day, without feeling broken. It was spring now, four months after her death. It surprised me, even shocked me, and made me feel quite sick because of the violence of the fact my sister could be dead, and I could be OK, as if I'd suddenly swept my arm across a table laid with cups and saucers, smashing them all in the process but finding a certain beauty in the emptiness of the clear table and the crash of everything being broken and gone. Finding that I could actually be OK for a whole day was a terrible, shocking relief.

I tried to work out ways to control how sad I felt, so that the pain didn't just suddenly jump up and kick me in the guts out of nowhere. For a few weeks, in late spring, I saw a grief therapist. Of course, because this was while the country was still locked down against the coronavirus, I could not see her IRL but instead by weekly Zoom meetings. She had a reassuring face and wore little gold earrings and neat white shirts, talking to me from a sitting room where she sat deep on a big sofa, a mahogany table beside her. Although I didn't ask her, I imagined she must be at home and I wanted to step inside it since it looked so comfortable, so safe, and so secure. I talked to her from my bedroom, from where I could hear Evangeline talking to Dolly in the garden, and Dash and Lester sitting on the landing outside my room, building wooden train tracks. Sometimes the children would fight, or Dash would hammer on my door, or our dog Pablo would bark, all off screen, obviously, and I'd see the therapist vaguely registering another life beyond my face, although she never said anything. Compared to the inside of her home I saw on the screen, I felt chaotic. Once, when I was talking to her, my chair broke so that I suddenly toppled over. Perhaps this feeling of chaos was intensified by the churning feeling of rage leading to helplessness that my weekly sessions precipitated in me. That was the place at which I started each appointment with her. I was angry about the emotional turmoil that death had brought into my life and which I was battling with every day. I had tried hard to make my life organized or at the very least to work in its disorganized way. I am naturally a disorganized person and I like excess – it's why I have five children and I would never choose order over excitement and strong motion – but even so I had tried to manage things so that my life worked well. In pursuing my own course, I had organized my life as much as I could, but there will always be a horrifically messy top drawer in the kitchen full of very old Sellotape, dog flea treatment, plaiting bands, children's vitamins, batteries, phone-charger cables with no plugs, broken sticks of chalk, a silver mug, some spurs, a Tupperware box with different size envelopes in it, a jam jar of Dash, Evangeline and Lester's first hair when I cut it, a letter about my tax code and some hairbrushes with bristles of different strengths. And in some sense this drawer is a bit like my life. I knew how to live in a state of organized mess, I suppose, but my sister's death really confused everything. It was like going to sleep in a room in which you knew where all the piles of books were and how to put your hands on a pair of socks or the shirt you wanted, only to wake up every morning to find that the space around you had been entirely ransacked, everything emptied out and upended and ripped and broken. Waking up and knowing my sister was dead felt a bit like having to remake my life again every day just so that I could get through the everyday: just so that I could get dressed and brush my teeth. And that made me feel very tired and also often very angry. I didn't want to be doing this work! I wanted to be living the messy, organized life I had created without having to remake it all the time. I could not see where the relief would come from. I could not see the point in having to reorganize everything every day.

'You just miss her, don't you? It just hurts a lot, the way you miss her, doesn't it?' the therapist said to me from inside her tidy and comfortable-looking house inside my screen. My face, beamed back to me through Zoom, looked grotesque: red and puffy and contorted, with snot running from my nose. She had asked me where the pain was and what it felt like.

What does the pain of missing your sister feel like? Where do you register that pain in your body? Can you explain what it feels like?

I could not control my face as I tried to explain the way the hurt really felt. The missing was like a physical pain which sat in my throat and my chest, and rang in my ears. It was like an actual physical disgust with the reality of her death and the way that it had forced me to reorganize all the spaces in my life to make room for the melancholy and longing and poignancy and guilt and confusion and raging anger that had taken over and claimed much bigger spaces than they would normally do. (Of course I am not saying that these things had not played a part in my life until my sister had died, because they had formed the texture of my entire life, but they had sat alongside joy, surprise, pleasure, fulfilment, desire too. But all the more difficult, hot feelings became a lot bigger after my sister died, so that they didn't just fill the room, they *were* the room.) Missing her was as though someone had scooped out the entire inside of my body so that often I felt I was walking around like a carcass of a being, just a body but not really there. Missing her was like trapdoors opening under me, sudden vertigo spinning me out, as if someone had gouged out my eyeballs and I'd never really see life in the same way again. It was like walking around with a highly contagious disease you didn't want anyone else to catch.

Missing her was the way I breathed and slept and walked and was. And I told the therapist that that sense of missing scared me. The enormity of the pain of missing scared me so much because it took over everything. Even when I tried to push the feelings away, they were always there, and I knew that in order to honour my sister I had to feel them, too.

Missing her and missing the conversation, the fights, the rows, the laughs, the connections, the understanding of what we were to one another as sisters and human beings, ran through every part of my life. When I thought of the fact that I could not talk to her, I felt as though I would vanish into nothing.

I was finding it impossible to think about death without seeing myself in combat with it. The knights were with me a lot of the time. They pulled me forward through the forest, when part of me wanted, still, to go backwards in time, back through the portal to her. My sister was alive recently enough to be able to imagine doing this. I could still turn around and touch the past although it was receding faster and faster as the world all around me changed too. I had not yet bowed down and surrendered. I was still at work with a clashing sword trying to fight. I was still maddened enough by death to think I could somehow beat it as it flashed all around me. You see how wild being close to death makes you feel? You see how confused loss makes you feel? When I tried to read books about death and grief, I often found that the stories there didn't reflect what I was feeling. The books themselves didn't either. So often they were dark grey or black, with the outline of winter leaves or bones on them. Most of the time I didn't feel grey, or black, and I didn't have the relief of feeling transparent. Inside me was a fizzy mess of furious, colliding colours that was always on the point of giving me a migraine.

Often, too, I felt as though I had bees under my skin. Until my sister died I had imagined that grief and the life that goes on after death – the life of those people who remain alive – would have been turned black, or at least a dull grey. It really wasn't the kind of colour I'd paint in my house, where I have green window frames in the kitchen, an orange colour round the washing machine where the dirty laundry is dumped, a turquoise cooker and a pink sitting room. Dash and Lester's room has more of the bright orange in it where I was using up the paint and their

bookshelves are vivid yellow. The bedroom Pete and I
sleep in is a strong green, plastered with paper covered in
almost emerald-coloured leaves, so that a sense of the outside comes in, even in the darkness of sleep. And what I
was finding since my sister died was that having been
taken close to death could also turn life inside out with
bright colours. Sometimes, as I have mentioned before, the
colours were so bright they felt totally blinding: the jewel-
bright orange of the wrapping paper and tinsel at Christmas;
the scorching red pain of the furnace; the luminous blue-
violet bluebell woods where the green of the trees seemed
so bright it hurt my eyes; the violent dark blue of the sky as
I sat challenging it to answer me. And the battle with death
was also making me feel, sometimes, bright pink with
energy.

I felt that pinkness of rage one afternoon, sometime during
the late spring, after lockdown was lifting a bit and a friend
arrived to sit, suitably distant, in the garden. She wasn't a
close friend, but someone I knew from my work as a journalist, whom I'd first met a decade before, on a press trip to
Italy. We'd remained in touch through the previous ten
years, sometimes sending each other book suggestions,
occasionally meeting at work events in London. She'd had
a child, a son who was five, and he arrived with her, tumbling out of the car after the drive from her home in Acton.
She was on the way to Bristol, to visit her sister, and she had
about her all the openness of the road, as if she'd been
gulping in the wide horizons as she drove.

'The world feels completely different,' she said, and I agreed. I'd wanted to hug her, but that was, what, illegal? So instead we danced around on the other side of the garden, waving, embarrassed by the new formality of a warm friendship. There were so many edges between us now, neither of us knew how to be. Her arrival had been a celebration – the first friend to arrive from London after lockdown! – and I had baked a cake that Evangeline had iced with bright yellow and brighter pink icing, pressing mint leaves into the sugar. She told me about lockdown in London, how it had been the hardest thing she had ever been through. She'd brought me a book of poetry and a box of tea.

After a while she said: 'How *are* you?'

There was a sincerity in her voice that scared me a bit. People say this because they want you to really tell them how you feel, but if you answer back: *I feel furious, sometimes insane, very lonely, confused by time and often unstable in place, and angry with other people and life, particularly angry with people with fully alive sisters and mothers*, it would be difficult to cope with. How can you move on from that and have a chatty conversation? So I just said something else that was true: 'I just really, really miss my sister.'

She looked at me and nodded, saying, 'I imagine, I imagine you do.' She said she'd never lost anyone close before.

'My husband's granny passed away. But I suppose that was different. I don't think I could cope without my sister,'

she replied, and in my head a very, very loud voice said to
this woman:

DON'T SAY IT.

Don't say what you're thinking, because I know exactly
what the sentence is that's about to come out of your mouth
and I do not want to hear it.

DON'T SAY IT.

But she couldn't hear the voice and so she went on: 'I
can't begin to imagine how you must feel. I can't imagine
what your loss must feel like. There's nothing like the bond
between sisters, is there? I really couldn't manage life without my sister. We're so close. I really could not cope
without her.'

She smiled a little and I heard Dash shouting at Lester in
another room, 'That's not FAIR!' as I concentrated on the
slice of pink and yellow cake on the chipped plate. I wanted
to take a knife and mash the piece of cake into the plate
and then smash the plate against the wall of my house
where the sun hit the cracks. I wanted to slap this woman
so hard in the face, but because I couldn't, instead I thought
hard about bright pink to contain the rage in front of me.

She didn't stay long after that and I was pleased I wasn't
able to hug her when she left. Instead, I just waved weakly

like a stupid clown from the other side of the garden. After-wards I gathered the plates and cups up from the table outside, stubbing my toe on the edge of a chair, dropping a knife on to the lawn and dumping the china in the sink with such ferocity a mug smashed. I pressed my hands against the edge of the sink and thought about the physical pain that the therapist had asked me to identify in my body, and I felt it now pressing in my throat. It came rushing down into my body even though I tried to stop it. I carried on clearing the table and as I picked up the pink and yellow cake I felt sobs racking through me, tears streaming on top of the cake, ruining the coloured icing.

When I stopped crying, and after the children were in bed, I walked out into the garden, looking for signs, for something to hang on to. There was nothing, just the empty garden and the sound of a child shouting in an upstairs bedroom. I kicked the end of my trainer into the gravel, angry that I'd wasted eggs and sugar and butter on a cake. When I looked down, there was a pebble, shaped like a perfect heart, lying directly beside the tip of my trainer. It was sandy-coloured and fitted right into the centre of my hand. I squeezed it and turned it over, feeling the warmth of it where it had just been sitting there, amongst thousands and thousands of other very old stones in the drive, waiting for me to find it. At that moment I remembered standing outside my house, two years before, when I had been feel-ing very sad and overwhelmed. I had called my sister while standing barefoot on the stones in the drive.

'Put a stone in your pocket. Just find a little stone and put it in your pocket as something to hold on to, Clo,' she had said, telling me that men who had been soldiers in the Second World War had sometimes carried stones in their pockets to hold on to.

I squeezed the stone and turned back to the house, where there was honeysuckle growing up the edge of a drainpipe beside the rosemary I had planted at the same time I had been speaking to my sister about pebbles. ('Plant lots of rosemary. You can't go wrong planting rosemary. You can't overdo it with rosemary,' she had also said.) Fat striped bees moved lazily now between the horns of the honeysuckle, and behind it I noticed a crimson dicentra I had planted two years before. It had never flowered before and I'd thought that it had died, if I thought about it at all. Now, though, a single heart hung from the bush. I had a long-distant memory of having been told that dicentra was magic and could be planted to ward off witches. I went into the sitting room where there was a book on the folklore and meaning of plants that I'd got the year before from my friend who was a gardener. I had not seen her for a few years but had then started seeing her a lot, walking around her garden with her as we talked about birth and loss and important things like that, and she had given me the book. I'd had an idea that she might teach me about gardening as she knew so much and had such an easy way of discussing it. Talking to her about plants never turned into the long lecture it can so often feel like when other people tell me how to garden. I had wanted to read the book and process it seriously, and I had started going to see her regularly and had done some gardening with her. She had a small golden wheelbarrow that Dash and Lester liked to fill with weeds and then push around. She certainly had a lot of rosemary growing too. But then very suddenly, two months before my sister died, she had also died, and I had not read any more of her book.

Now for the first time since either my friend or my sister had died, I pulled the book out and sat with it on my lap.

All parts of the plant are poisonous, although mortality is very rare. Symptoms of **dicentra** poisoning may include intense sleepiness, vomiting, convulsive movements, coma and unequally dilated pupils.

I closed the book and walked back into the kitchen, thinking of the woman telling me she *could not cope* if *her* sister died, as if there was a choice. As I started stacking the plates in the dishwasher, scraping icing sugar and half-eaten pieces of cake into the bin, I wondered whether, if I had decorated it with dicentra rather than mint leaves, the symptoms it would have given her might have opened her mind to what it can feel like to have to *cope* with a dead sister. I thought about how I sometimes felt violent with anger towards people who didn't understand or who were in that strange place of not yet having had to understand. I had so much anger inside me I felt dizzy, and maybe it was this dizziness that made me break the tip of the spout of my favourite blue teapot, cutting the edge of my thumb on the small blue chip as I reached into the plug hole to fish it out.

My blood was bright as it dropped into the white of the sink, and when I looked up, there was a gold cup I had bought in a charity shop in Gloucester with my sister and it was on the floor, spinning around.

Later that night, I put the heart-shaped stone on the table by my bed, beside a wooden bear that had once been in one of the children's stockings. I had told Evangeline, 'When you cannot bear things any longer, you hold on to the bear.' Alongside it was a small collection of Madonnas and a string of glass beads I have had since I was about twenty. I found these beads in my bedroom when I was a student and I don't know where they came from but I feel less of myself if they are not near me in some way. (My children have become accustomed to me saying, 'Where are my beads? Where are my beads?' if I lose them, as though a string of the most precious diamonds has been taken from me.) On the bedside table I also had a small metal talisman in the shape of Jesus that I'd bought with my sister in a junk market in Cirencester one year before I found the heart-shaped stone in the drive. It was the same market we used to go to as children, taking pocket money to spend on old teddy bears, broken lockets, farm toys, as if our childhood had been extremely old-fashioned, although it had not felt like it at the time. I squeezed the heart-shaped stone and the wooden bear as I thought about the fact that we had been alive together so recently, and that seemed like a magic trick in itself. I could see too that what I was doing with all these special little objects was creating a shrine.

The stone, the bear, the Christ and some photographs and a small yellow reed box of worry people on my bedside table were offerings that I found reassuring, even as the children hid under the table and knocked them over. The shrine of hard little objects were things to clasp, when the caverns of loss opened up and life felt as if it was sliding out of reach.

I had a photograph beside my bed of my sister sitting with Dash on a hill near her home. Their blond hair was blowing in the wind, and my then two-year-old son and my now dead sister were laughing at one another. I propped the photograph up behind the shrine of little pieces and kept it there for a few nights. After a few more nights, I turned it over and put it face down on the pile of books by my bed. My sister had died in early winter and now it was late spring, so this was two seasons since I had last seen my sister alive and I still could not look at photographs of her without a caustic pain hurting me. It was still better not to look.

Chapter 6

So Dazzling and So Awful

There were a lot of exceptionally hot days in the spring and early summer and the children were always at home as the schools were closed. I tried to make them read every day or learn their times tables but most of the time I found it impossible. They shouted at me and ran out of my reach when I said it was time to study, and often before I even said it too. I returned to the stories of the knights, as a way to ground myself. Remembering how Gawain and Lancelot moved forwards inside their myths helped me keep going when I felt like turning back.

I wasn't sure if the feeling I had of tired, bored, mashed head was the pandemic or my personal grief, since both had completely changed my life in every way, even while it still looked the same. Everything was old and yet new, but I was aware this wasn't my experience alone. Sometimes it felt as if we were all, collectively, standing on the table in the middle of a room we knew well and seeing it from a completely altered angle and in an entirely different light.

'O Captain! my Captain!' we all called to one another vaguely through the mist.

Hot days dripped into one another and the children ran in and out of the house, spreading puddles from the paddling pool and dried grass picked up on their bare feet. In the evenings, I walked into the garden and tried to convince myself I was interested in gardening. I found it monotonous and frustrating. Nothing seemed to happen that I could really see. Even cutting off the dead heads of roses, which I thought might have been melancholic and lyrical, bored and irritated me. Very occasionally, I knelt down at dusk, pushing my fingers into the earth, wondering what I was supposed to be doing with all these weeds and plants that now needed my attention like my children did, but which I ignored, even more than the children.

Yet despite the fact I neglected the garden, something had worked there. Lettuces and courgettes grew in the ground that Jimmy and Teyte had dug in the spring. This seemed like some kind of miracle as I had done nothing to help these small plants.

If I had hoped to find some kind of meaning in the earth, I was disappointed as I scratched around with a child-size gardening fork that bent in the dry soil. Sometimes I'd ask Dash or Evangeline to come and garden beside me, imagining we might have a sweet moment where they picked their first courgette or dug up a worm which we might be able to turn into a home-school project. Actually, they were as perplexed by what to do with the soil and the weeds as I was, and would quickly run away saying it was boring. I'd agree, abandoning my fork and half-picked lettuces to find Jimmy to make him roll a cigarette for me.

Gardening was supposed to make me feel grounded. People kept telling me on Instagram to just put my hands into the soil and that would make me feel better about all the grief that was around but the frustration I felt when I made myself do any kind of gardening made me more aware of my stupid human failings than I had almost all year. It was the same anger I'd felt when someone had told me that my sister would quietly reveal herself in surprising ways. I wanted her back noisily and I didn't want any more fucking surprises. Also I wanted to feel less a part of this earth, not more grounded to it. At my most optimistic I felt that perhaps learning about great sorrow and loss could almost be an act of daring. I thought again about the girl who'd sat in the garden and told me *I can't imagine what your loss must feel like* and the messages and letters which said that my loss was *unimaginable*. I wasn't just imagining it but looking right at it and feeling it and waking up while cradling it every day, tasting it, wearing it, breathing it. And I thought the daring bit could be in seeing what lay beyond the loss and what might happen after I'd passed through it, if that ever happened. Maybe that would show me something about life and being alive that people who had not experienced loss – those who were living in that apparently secure yet also horrifically precarious place of never having grieved – did not know about. And there could be value in that, although it was also clear that there was a lot of hard work involved. Dash could not learn his times tables by simply sitting and staring at a list of numbers. He had to practise the numbers. Accepting the endless absence of someone you love very much is a bit like this: it takes practice and hard work to put it into your mind in such a way that it becomes acceptable to your brain and then almost second nature. The shock of loss I had felt in the first months after my sister was dead had changed into something I could fathom every day. I no longer felt as if I was poisoned but I still struggled to accept the fact of her death. But for the first time since her death I was also curious about the place I would get to when my brain could comprehend this.

Maybe it could be a daring and exciting place to get to.

That was the most optimistic thing I could think about my sister's death. I would learn about life. I'd walk around the garden watching the sunlight changing on the grass, ignoring the dead heads of roses, and imagine that there might be something I could learn which was golden and valuable. And then I'd think: there, that's optimistic. And I'd feel excited about it and wonder where Jimmy was so that I could go and smoke one of his roll-ups to celebrate. But in that moment of feeling happy, something confusing like a crest falling would happen inside me and I'd think: But, you stupid fucking fool, you'd swap all the golden knowledge in the world just to be able to go back in time, with your sister, to that place of precarious ignorant security where you were before.

And then I'd feel so depressed I'd have to go and find Jimmy anyway as smoking was a way of softening the edges until all there was was a revolting taste of dirty tobacco in my mouth and a lovely nicotine buzz in my blood.

But the realization that there was value in loss that had felt unbearable was sort of liberating in ways too.

One of the very worst things I could imagine had happened.

And yet life was going on.

As I said, dazzling.

And also so awful.

As the ground heated and baked, and days and days rolled on and on with that strange sort of mid-August-nothing flavour, I realized I had stopped talking to my dead sister. She never answered, anyway, and instead I just heard my own voice, taunting me that I was being stupid and sentimental. I stopped looking for signs or grasping at the idea I'd seen her in a leaf that floated down and fell through an open car window as I sat in a supermarket car park, or in a beam of sunlight piercing my blinds. It was just a beam of sunlight. Once I was walking down the road with Evangeline on her bicycle when a black cat suddenly walked past us and I felt an urge to say to Evangeline, *Look, that's her!* But it really was just a black cat. Symbols didn't work and things that had seemed mystical were normal. When I talked to my sister, there was total silence apart from a loud ringing noise in my ears.

*

Other voices were very, very important though. Everything about Pete's voice has always mattered to me a lot. I always want to hear what he is saying to me. Even when we are fighting, I still want him to fuck me and to hear his voice in my ear. He is the person I want to talk to before anyone.

And I spoke on the phone to my dad and stepmother often. I might even have talked to them daily. We certainly communicated in some way every day – email or WhatsApp or a comment on Instagram – if we didn't have an actual conversation. I really loved this. I have never had difficulty talking to my father and stepmother but it was as though death had shown me a new, special value in keeping them close: like shining a bright flashlight into a cupboard and finding a whole array of beautiful clothes you have not worn for a while.

It was also important to me to hear their voices so that I knew they had not died. I worried about this all the time, but I could also see that something important was happening: new areas of my soul, new places where my love could go were opening up around me. It also felt crucial to communicate with them how much I loved them. Can you imagine something worse than the person you love dying without you having told them you loved them? I started doing this with my friends, too. It's easy to say, 'Love you' at the end of a phone conversation but try saying, 'I love you.' You might hear the silence after you say that, or a hurried, 'Love you too.' There is a special, direct power in *I love you*. And also, since my sister had died I wanted certain people, who I loved, to really know it. I wanted them to know it until I had bored them with telling them. So that there was not a fraction of space for doubt. That's important.

Because one of the other things death had brought into my life was guilt and regret. I wanted to be able to go back and tell her again and again and again and again and again and again how much I loved her. I wanted to tell her again.

The inability to do that was a horrible feeling like a rat gnawing away at the soles of my feet. These things not said burrowed into me and settled in dirty places inside me.

I should have spent more time with her when we were both alive.

I should have said YES! not I'm on a deadline when she'd messaged me a month before she died saying Meet for lunch?

I should have cancelled that meeting and taken her to another chemotherapy session in the summer before she died.

I shouldn't have been angry about that conversation.

I should have not got cross.

I should have done more.

I should have been more present.

I should have been kinder.

I should not have argued.

I should have stayed the night, that time, so many times, when she said, 'Stay the night? Come on! Stay the night!'

I should have been different.

I should have been a different person.

I should have been a better person and I should have died not her.

Death had taken her from me and filled parts of my brain up with regret for the things not said, the conversations unfinished, the time not shared. I wanted to relive the last moments with her, too, when I tried to express a whole lifetime of love for one another in a few moments. I tried to console myself with the idea that I would always have been left with a desire for more. We all might want one more conversation, but how can there ever, ever be enough? This was the thing that made me scream, when I was walking alone in a distant place so I could make a noise no one should hear.

One day in therapy, the therapist, whose face and calm, consoling voice I'd come to crave as she smiled at me, slightly, from a squashy sofa in her comforting home, asked me:
     'If you could say anything to her and you could hear anything back from her, what would it be?'
     I looked at her, and for a split second I could see my sister, as if she too was on Zoom, her face patient but persisting, waiting for her answer. I wanted to reach into the screen and touch her, and in that longing I felt my shoulders falling and a familiar pressure in my chest, a tightening around my neck, a silencing of my voice as that feeling pushed at me, pushing me and pushing me so that I couldn't speak, and I couldn't hear for the ringing in my head, and I was ashamed of the squeaking, whimpering sound I was making. We sat like that for some time, in between two screens, my head

bowed as tears splashed on to my keyboard because I could not speak for the pain of feeling my inability to say the thing to my sister which I wanted to say. There was noise somewhere downstairs of one of my children crying, but it was not for me that that child was reaching out.

Eventually I choked out the only answer that ever mattered.

'If I could see my sister I would say, I want you to know that I love you with all my heart and I want to know that you loved me.'

I said it again and again to the therapist, repeating it until the silence in my ears had gone.

Afterwards, as I looked back up from the keypad to the screen, to that kind, comforting face, I realized I had started breathing again. And she was soothing me and comforting me as she might a small child, telling me that it was so obvious, it was *so* obvious, the love that was between us. When I could fully speak again, the therapist asked me another question.

'If you could hear your sister answering you, what would she say?'

'She would say that she loves me, and that she knows beyond doubt that I love her too.'

She knows and I know.

There's nothing else.

In the middle of the summer, as lockdown lifted, there was something important I had to do.

'Please, do it soon. Do it immediately,' my stepmother said to me.

I had been putting it off for different reasons, but I knew I needed to go to London to speak to my sister's oncologist. I had met him often with my sister and spoken to him after she had died. He told me about the gene my sister had carried that might have caused her death, and he wanted me to consider having a test, to see if I carried it too. This was the thing my stepmother wanted me to urgently do.

I felt very cross with life that I was stepping back into the waiting room where we had sat together, eating the free biscuits they left for patients waiting. Her oncologist was from Guildford, and he was slightly bald and very direct. He wasted no words. After we came out from the first appointment with him my sister had said she really fancied him and I had agreed with her.

Now I was sitting in his office alone in front of him, without her, because he wanted to tell me about what the genetic testing really meant, but also, I realized, as he started talking, because he just wanted to talk to me about her. He told me she was an unforgettable life force and that he was thankful for having met her since he wasn't sure he'd ever know someone like her again.

'I was proud to be her doctor,' he said in that direct way I had noticed the first time I met him when he had been telling my sister and me how many years she might be able to live for. 'She inspired me. Being her doctor has made me redouble my efforts in cancer research, to try to help other people.'

As he spoke, I became aware of the fact that I was sitting up very straight in the high-backed chair, as if I was in a job interview, preparing myself to try to get all the conversation right and so pass the test. We talked about cancer and the life my sister had lived with cancer and the life that we as her family had lived around her. I told him about the ways I missed her and that there were things I felt so guilty about: the times I had not been able to be there for her which I regretted so much, and which I'd never have back. And he looked at me closely, in his direct way, and then he said there would always be a difference between what you feel you can do to help someone, and what you can actually do.

He said: 'After decades of experience in oncology I know it's absolutely normal for people to think, I wish I had done more. It's a normal part of the adjustment from a world in which we have that person, to a world in which we have that person in memory. A thinking, loving person will always feel like this and it's part of facing death, I believe. Our world doesn't always let us do the things or live in the way we wish it might have done. But that does not diminish anything, it doesn't diminish any love you had for each other which exceeded appointments or practical issues. And hear me when I say to you that everything you say to me about feeling guilt and regret, mixed with your loss and love, absolutely resonates with thousands of stories I have heard from other families facing a loss as great as yours. She spoke about you so much; she spoke of her family all the time. She loved you so much. And when she died, it was in a place free from fear.'

I breathed out, my shoulders slumping, my torso slumping too. Relief rushed into me, since this man, who had
known the inside of my sister's body in such detail, who
had known her DNA and been able to read her genetic
make-up down to individual particles, including those particles that killed her (and which, he told me later, I did not
carry), was at last able to give me reassurance and an
answer, one I'd been hunting for and straining to listen out
for with every particle of my own being.

But what was surprising, and you might say sometimes
exhausting, was that that reassurance didn't stop me looking for my sister. Even as I left the clinic, stepping out into
the grey street under a sharp blue sky, past a glare of bright
pink geraniums in a window box, I immediately started
searching again. The search wasn't over. It was getting dark,
taxis swooping along, the occasional flash of a red bus, and
as I walked through Soho I was taken aback by a meat-
refrigeration lorry unloading frozen boxes into the back of
a supermarket. There was a novelty to seeing the streets and
the cars and shops, mostly closed, but still there, which was
exciting after so many months of having been at home.

I was aware of everything and could feel everything,
time and sense moving through me as I walked into the
dusk. Shadows from the inside of a building cast a line of
little crucifixes of light on to the pavement that I tried not to
stand on. There was a sharpness to the early-evening light
which I don't think was just a result of having spent two
hours talking to a man who had studied my sister's genes,

but by the time I got to Oxford Street I felt as though I was spinning a bit, chasing and chasing after something I was not sure I could identify but which, if I had had to name, I might have described as a sort of lightness. It wasn't cold but I had an overwhelming desire to go into a shop and buy an expensive new piece of clothing. I wanted to wrap myself in something comforting that might also be coloured tangerine orange or vivid pink.

Straight away I found myself in the kind of shop I don't usually go to: tiny trench coats with floral lining hanging in sets of three, satin dresses like cold water moving slightly as I passed them, little slips of coloured silk folded into piles of vests. There, an intense and beautiful girl with brown, extremely shiny hair and long limbs was folding skinny scarves into knots. I couldn't see anywhere to pay and I immediately started sweating. Not because of the lack of till, but because it was so hot. Every place I moved in this store felt as if hot air was blowing at me like a hairdryer.

I thought that it wasn't a shop for me but then I reached out and picked up a pink cardigan with a pink and white striped edging, a bit like an American bomber jacket with threads of silver glitter woven into the material. It had green flecks in the fabric and several different shades of pink decorating it, all very hot. It was dense and strong so that it felt as if it could almost stand up on its own. I thought this might be a good thing if I was having one of those moments when I felt as if I might fall over, that *gravitational collapse*, or when my shoulders just gave way, things that still happened to me quite often out of the blue even though I was into the third season since my sister's death. There was a pattern on it that I didn't really notice properly until later, when I realized it was cherries. It was the only cardigan like that in the shop and it was also half-price and the perfect size.

It was dark by the time I left the shop and I was completely pleased with the bomber jacket cardigan because it was exactly the kind of extravagant and colourful piece of clothing my sister would have worn. It wasn't what I would usually wear so, if I thought about it, I had an uncomfortable feeling the cardigan was wearing me, but I put this aside and instead just felt the flow of people and faces walking towards me, my eyes darting over them all, searching for only one person. I had walked to all the places she had walked to. I had sat in the waiting room where she had sat many times. I had walked down the shopping street where she spent money. Surely I must be about to walk round in a circle and bump into her? The traffic that passed me in the street seemed to be incredibly close, almost excitingly so, and at any moment I felt I might just be able to step into the path of one of these impactful red buses as it whooshed past me and took me onwards quickly to death. I felt myself glancing behind as a siren suddenly went off, a shrill, engulfing sound, and I was surprised all these people walking past me didn't hear it too and jump a little. I was also shocked that the lady walking towards me holding a small girl by the wrist didn't pull the child closer to her because of the siren. Didn't she care if the little girl was swept away to death too? But then I suddenly realized this siren was the one in my head, except I'd got better at turning it down. Now the shape it made in my mind was more like this:

WHEREAREYOUWHEREAREYOU
WHEREAREYOUWHEREAREYOUWHEREAREYOU
WHEREAREYOUWHEREAREYOU.

I could dial it down to a feeling more like tinnitus than a siren. But even so I was still looking amongst the sea of faces streaming towards me for her: for my sister. It was getting darker and I wondered if I would be wrong to stay in the city for a bit longer: postpone going back to my children because of the sense of freedom and almost exhilaration that being out in the dark streets, my feet carrying me over the concrete pavements, gave me.

I continued walking but tried to work out how long I could stay before I must get back, and what times the trains might be running. And my brain started churning, all the thoughts and words and train times and images of my children's disappointed little faces waiting for me at the window, confusing my mind, since they did this sometimes. Sometimes my children sat at the window, staring out into the darkness of the fields around our house and the one road, waiting and watching for me to come home, which now worried me a great deal, since what would happen to them and their hearts if that car crash I imagined so often really did happen to me? These jumbled and mixed-up thoughts were like the milk my sister and I used to put into a jam jar and then shake and shake and shake until it changed from liquid into butter. The churning inside of my brain felt as if it had changed from milk to butter in the same way and suddenly when I looked up from the pavement at more people and then beyond them, further down the street, my sister was walking towards me.

Golden, tall, shimmering, crackling white-blonde hair a halo of light around her iridescent skin, cheekbones jutting, eyes like dark bolts, her shoulders wide under a black coat with golden buttons fastened from her throat downwards, my sister was moving slowly towards me in the darkness. The line of her vision was over my shoulder and since she wasn't looking at me, I couldn't catch her eye, but even so, I could not breathe, I could not hear, I could not feel – not my hands, nor most of my body. I could feel my heart but nothing else. She was close enough to touch and I knew I had been right and her death certificate had been wrong just as it had reminded me that this might be the case: 'WARNING: CERTIFICATE IS NOT EVIDENCE OF IDENTITY.'

She had not died. Perhaps she had moved to the furthest part of the country or perhaps indeed to another part of the world, or perhaps she had just hidden somewhere really quite close by but equally invisible and now she was returning. She walked directly towards me through the dark city, golden woman, precious pearl, all her light and love around her because she was back, she had not died, she had not gone, she had not left, she was back and I had found her.

When the tall woman with bleached blonde hair and shiny pale skin in the long black coat passed me I found I could feel my hands again but my heart was beating too fast and my breathing was shallow so I knew that waiting to get a late train home was not something I should do. I was vulnerable and it would not be good to walk around in this state. My face was completely wet.

All the stars were out when I drove back into the yard at home two hours later and the sky around them was black as anything.

Chapter 7

Two Treacherous Edges and Ponies in the Dark

The thought that I had imagined seeing my sister turned me backwards on a fork in the path where I had thought I was walking forwards. I found myself returning to a place in the forest that I thought I'd already passed through. It wasn't like the time in the spring when I thought about her almost incessantly, when she was tapping on the inside of my eyelids, but in late summer I felt obsessed by her and by death all over again. I had been trying to walk myself through the year by imagining myself as a knight on a quest looking for meaning in her death, but halfway through the year I felt defeated. There was still such a long way to go.

I knew Galahad was with me, but I had hoped that soon I would be able to ride without him beside me. In late summer I realized that the path through the forest, where the frost is undisturbed and there's no one else's track to follow, is crooked and that often it crosses back on itself. I'd feel as if I was making progress then find myself, quite suddenly, in a dark clearing surrounded by the spiked thorns of a sharp bramble patch. I felt as if I was having to walk the same path again and again, going over ground I'd already covered. And the ground I went back to was always the hard places: where the forest was darkest, where the thorns were most spiked and where I was most afraid of what might lie in wait.

I have told you that in the weeks immediately after my sister died I had felt a desire to become nothing. This was in the days when I was on the rack and could no longer write or even sometimes talk. While in my deepest heart I knew I wasn't going to 'commit' anything, a desire simply to no longer exist was strong.

That desire for oblivion had mostly left me in the spring, but at the end of August, those flat long days when the brightness of 8 December 2019, the last day my sister was still alive on this planet, subsided into the past, I found that desire for non-existence returning. I often saw my life stretching ahead of me and it didn't seem possible that I could manage to live through all those long days when my sister was not there too. I kept this secret to myself. I didn't tell Pete, and of course I couldn't tell my children about my own wish to die. I didn't tell anyone.

I started wondering about different ways that a state of nothingness could be achieved and thought of the train

accident. Although I feel quite possessive of it, since it's absolutely mine and makes me who I am, which is of course neurotic, anxious and regularly depressed, but also brave, resilient and strong, it is not something I would wilfully choose to pass on to my children.

It was much, much easier to vanish into the reaches of a substance. In the evenings immediately after my sister died, I wanted to drink red wine, soft like velvet to hide within, and in the summer that feeling returned very strongly. I wanted to take the edge off how tired the feeling of missing my sister made me. I bought some Valium from someone who used to sell me ecstasy when I was younger, and also little dark bottles of CBD oil with a 1:1 concentration of THC. I was smoking heavily too, at first cigarettes I borrowed from Jimmy and then I started buying packets of my own. A little brown trail of tobacco snaked over the black slate work surfaces in the kitchen sometimes, which was revolting, but it was worth it for the sense of detachment that came from sitting outside on my own as nicotine worked through my veins. Tending to a little addiction became a way of tending to myself.

Sometimes I felt as if I was operating between two sharp edges which were both equally perilous. Smoking and taking Valium or drinking red wine, or imagining the feeling of stepping off the railway bridge, were a way of blunting the edges, and having a rest from the quest that was perpetually tugging at me, even when I was just looking after the children or driving to the shops. No one can deny that there are moments, three glasses in, when red wine is the most

perfect painkiller. And Valium too. It just knocks the emotion out of things. Liberation from all these great big feelings
in a little blue pill. I don't want you to think I was taking it
all the time, because I really wasn't and anyway, even if I
had wanted to, I don't have a good enough supplier to take
it constantly. A regular GP will never give you enough Valium. I just kept it for quiet little moments when I needed to
be at home and in the house looking after the children, but
my mind needed to depart. Missing her was a distracting
feeling to live with. It got everywhere, the way glitter does,
and was difficult to remove, like chewing gum, that time
Evangeline got it in her hair. I wanted to feel her as a being
that was close to me but not inside me. I wanted to feel
more joy, because this was after all my one perfect life, and
I wanted to dislodge the feeling that when I felt joy I was
somehow betraying her.

In late August we were away, staying for a long weekend in
a house with a river running close to it. It was sparsely fur-
nished in that reassuring way holiday houses can be. There
were no superfluous ornaments the children might break,
lamps they might knock over or mirrors they might kick a
ball into. It was hot and I felt as relaxed as I had felt all year.
Each night I cooked supper for Pete and the children and
tried to put away the thought that the old-fashioned phone
might ring in the hallway, the lamp might flicker and my
sister would be there. Instead, I tried to relax into the feeling
that the holiday was a place that I was inhabiting, and that I
was permitted – encouraged even – to be happy for whole

days inside it. There were days, lying beside the river, Dash and Lester making so much noise throwing sand from the bank at one another, when I felt bored and frustrated, which is what motherhood often makes me feel, and when I wanted to be somewhere else, alone, so instead I would concentrate on the idea that my sister would have done anything to be there. I also tried to resist the urge I have always had to furiously record absolutely every moment of the children's lives in photographs. It comes from a fear that I am losing something important all the time, a feeling that's especially acute around my children. I wanted to make myself hold the present moment with a lighter touch and not grab on to it, afraid that it would vanish.

When I took the children to a small sweetshop near the river, I had to stop myself looking for signs of my sister. On a high shelf behind the till was a line of jars with sweets in them, and beside them, a plastic horse. I wanted to reach over the till and grab the plastic horse as a sign my sister had been there, somehow watching me and reminding me. I had to tell myself that it was just a small plastic horse. That it was not her, or anything to do with her. And that that was OK. At other times I had to stop myself from thinking I could call her to speak to her about all the things that had been going wrong in my head because she had died, and remind myself, quietly, that I could not do that any more, because she had died.

On the last day of the weekend, I went out to the river alone with Dash to try to stop him making so much noise. The lack of furnishings in the rented house was relaxing in terms of nothing being broken, but because there were few carpets on the wooden floors, it was very noisy with Dash in it.

There was a tall rock on one bank, where the water was waist-deep, where he could climb up and jump at me, as I stood, arms out, waiting for him. He jumped in again and again and again, until his teeth were chattering and his sun-browned skin looked as though he had been oiled. I was talking to him about my sister and how proud she would be to see him jumping and swimming. He smiled at me as he got ready to jump again; then, hurling himself at me, he said, 'She is a blur,' and this shocked me. He had talked about her often. He was five when she died. Her imprint would weaken. He would never know her as an adult. How could this be? I could not think of it, so instead we walked up the river as far as we could together, until the banks narrowed and we were just scrambling over rocks with water running between them. We could not swim in this stretch of the river and the greenery that hung all around was very bright and close. Dash said the rocks looked like dinosaur bones and there was a relief in this: the sense that the river would keep running, however much a heart hurt, because being five and jumping off a rock into cold river water again and again was all that mattered at that moment. He had made me feel alive inside a small diamond that was the present, a place I realized I wanted to be more often. When we drove home later that evening, the sun was sharp and bright, and we passed through tunnels that took us from the dark then straight back out into piercing sunlight. Driving from light to dark and back again in such swift succession was shocking but as we went I started to trust the sense that the brightness of the sky would always return.

In the autumn people started moving around a lot more than they had in the previous months. Pete went to America for his work and I spent two months on my own with the children, who started school, a place they hadn't been since March. I was on my own in the house again for long hours in the daytime. I wrote or stood at the table eating handfuls of raisins or played with the cats or folded laundry, or sometimes just sat in the kitchen staring tediously into nothing. Something was different. I felt different. Not better, and indeed sometimes a lot worse, but different.

I have said that I had stopped talking aloud to my sister; it was a habit I'd not dropped entirely but I hated the ringing silence and the voice that didn't reply and the endless searching for symbols which might mean nothing but into which I was trying to invest significance. In the autumn, I quietly came to realize that she might be there if I stopped trying to pull her towards me.

When you go out into a field to catch a pony in the dark, it's easier to see it if you stop trying to look directly at it or figure out what the shapes are in the darkness. If you look to the side of where you think the looming figure of the pony might be across the darkness of the field, sometimes it appears much more clearly. The magnificence of its shape reveals itself to you when you are not straining for something you cannot see.

Without being aware of it, I stopped looking for my sister. I didn't look at her photographs very often and I definitely did not look at any video of her. I stopped reading her letters and emails, texts, WhatsApp and Facebook messages and instead I started looking for ponies.

When I was outdoors, usually with animals, the shape death had made in my life seemed to change. No longer petrol blue and very tiring, almost threatening, to be around, instead it became the colourful shape of my life and the lives all around mine. In that way, I stopped noticing it.

At first, I wasn't really aware of this. Up until this point, nine months after my sister's death, I had had to make a firm and concerted effort to will myself into the present and to make myself available to my children, to be in the room with Pete. Except when I had sex, of course. Sex is the moment when you can empty your brain of everything but the absolute clear present moment. Sex is a whole house in my head, so when it's happening I can vacate everyday life and just be there instead.

However, as I said, Pete was away so there was no clear shining sex to empty my brain, and perhaps that was why I was able to find the horses, because they could occupy all my feelings and a big space in my mind too.

One weekend the rain did not let up all day and all night. I made slices of jam toast for the children and stood at the windows looking out. It was a continual sheet and even stepping outside the house for a few moments meant I was soaked to my pants. Because Pete was away, the idea of a whole weekend inside the house with Dash and Lester shouting for Lego or cups of milk made my head feel a bit glitchy so I spoke to my friends, Bill and Sally.

They live in the next village to ours and I had started to get to know them during the year. I had first met Sally a year before, about six months before my sister died, when she had arrived at our house and asked if she could leave a pony overnight in our field. When I say 'our field' that sounds big and important but actually it's just a tiny square of grass with a fence around it the size of some people's back garden. It is big enough for a pony to be in overnight but not to live in. Sally had arrived at our house in the darkness leading a chocolate-coloured pony with a golden mane. The pony's mane shone in the moonlight as golden as Sally's hair. I knew exactly who Sally was and although I had never spoken to her I had often wanted to. She wore tight black jeans and a top tucked into them with sequins shaped like a rose on the back. I knew she was a traveller and was married to the big traveller called Bill who drove a pickup and also sometimes trotted past our house on his cart. They kept ponies in the back garden of their semi-detached house, and sometimes tethered on the verge outside that house. There were chickens in their drive and often a green, yellow and red painted wagon, although the vehicles they had changed regularly, and the horses too. I often saw Bill and Sally, driving their horse and cart along the main road close to another village nearby where I'd drive to the Co-op for milk and sweets for the children. I would drive past them in my car, gripping the steering wheel as I tried to stare at them and their horse and cart but also keep one eye on the road.

When we first moved to the house I had bought a little grey pony called Trigger, who I drove in a cart when the children were all babies. Sometimes I noticed Bill looking at Trigger as he drove past me in his pickup. Bill and I still did not talk to one another although I was pleased when he started nodding at me when he saw me on my cart.

By the time my sister had died I had had to sell Trigger. Pete had had a bad accident in a terrorist scare and had broken both his legs very badly. That was in 2017 and Lester was a baby. For a time, Pete was in a wheelchair and we were not sure if he would walk again. It was impossible for me to keep a driving pony fit and help Pete learn to walk, and look after the small children and write my second book and have some rational thoughts too. So I'd sold Trigger back to the woman I bought him from, and although I didn't have a driving pony we did always have some ponies which I kept in a paddock I rented down by the village green. (I dream that one day we will have a field of our own – we all need things to dream about, don't we?)

Anyway, Bill is a big, big man with tattoos on his arms and across his hands and Sally has a faraway look on her face, and their horses were always beautiful: black and white Gypsy ponies or buckskin colts and dark brood mares they kept in a big area of rough open ground near to an industrial estate. Evangeline had started to go to a gymnastics club in a hangar on the industrial estate, and I could assuage the boredom of waiting outside the club for her to finish lessons looking at their horses tethered opposite the hangar.

After that night when Sally and I stood leaning over the gate in the moonlight looking at her horse in my little field, she had become my friend. Bill would wave at me when we passed in our cars, and then he started driving his pony over to our yard to talk. Bill and Sally liked chatting. They laughed a lot as we stood smoking together. They made jokes about everything and were open about everything.

I liked talking to them about horses and they taught me lots of new things I hadn't known before. Sally has a presence that's both absolutely there, connected to you, but also gently distant enough to feel relaxed with anything you talk about to her. They are proud to be travellers and I liked being able to ask them a lot of questions about their lives and how they lived and everything they knew about horses. They collected animals and often Bill would arrive with a ferret in his pocket or a puppy in the palm of his big hand.

Bill's sister had died some years before and he wanted to talk about her to me. He was the first person I'd met all year who I could talk to so openly about what it felt like to walk close to death. I could talk to him every day if I wanted about having a dead sister. There was consolation in that. A lot of people had looked scared or embarrassed by this kind of conversation and said things like, 'She'll always be in your heart' or, 'She'll always be with you,' but I didn't know what to do with those statements. I didn't feel as if my sister was with me. I didn't feel as if she was anywhere near me or anywhere at all most of the time. I absolutely didn't know where she was and when I arrived at month nine after her death I thought that maybe that was the best place I could get to – that was the *only* place I could get to. To simply accept that she had gone and silence the alarm in my head so that I could continue to walk through the days of my life even though she wasn't there, and even parts of me weren't there either.

Bill and Sally were important to this moment in my year because we started looking for horses together. It was a little project for me, I realized, with Pete away so much of the autumn. Weekends are long to fill in wet weather with small children but there was lots of space in Bill and Sally's pickup, and they never minded how much noise the children made; in fact they seemed to quite like an atmosphere of familial chaos. And they were generous with their time, so when another wet Saturday morning came around I piled Evangeline, Dash and Lester into the back seats of their pickup amongst the harnesses and puppies, and we drove around. (Jimmy and Dolly were too big to fit into the pickup and, anyway, looking for horses and talking about horses was of limited interest to them. They were at this time seventeen and twenty, with their own lives, quite separate from me, enlarging around them.)

Bill and Sally are horse dealers, so they know where all the yards are. We drove around, drinking lots of cans of Coke and stopping for chips they drenched in vinegar and salt, with country and western music playing on the radio. Sometimes, in between driving into a yard where we found nothing more than broken tractors or old trailers covered in tarpaulin wet with raindrops, we also talked about death and what it does to those left living who have come close to it. I could talk to Bill about these things. I could see that he had kept his eyes wide open and looked into the furnace, holding his face to the flames too.

He told me he had been changed by it completely, and that after his sister had died, for a long time he had wanted to die too. We'd been driving for a few hours when he first told me this, and we were waiting for an especially long time for some traffic lights to change by some slow roadworks.

'But I want to live now,' he said, reaching for another cigarette to smoke as the lights changed and we drove on.

In the back of the cab, Evangeline held a little white bulldog on her lap. Lester and Dash had gone to sleep.

We didn't talk about death any more that afternoon but drove down the A420 away from the downs on the edge of the village where we live, then on towards the outskirts of Swindon through the rain that fell in unrelenting sheets, windscreen wipers a hypnotic blur. Travellers know how to drive around suburbs and still find horses, because soon a field of Shetlands revealed itself through the rain and mist. Yes, the woman who had them did want to sell them. Yes, she was getting out of horses, too much work and neither of her sisters were interested. Yes, the ponies were all healthy, though a little neglected, for sure. Her ponies had matted manes and long feet but kind eyes and soft noses too; they walked into the horse box with almost a look of relief in their eyes, four Shetland ponies with brown and white hair.

We have a barn at home which until that winter had been used as a place to dump and store broken bicycles, old prams, wheelless skateboards, splintered fence posts, unthreading tennis rackets and other rubbish which I'd somehow struggled to throw away. During lockdown, the barn had found a purpose, since Jimmy pushed all the junk to one end to create an indoor skate room where he and his friends slammed backwards and forwards on skateboards, ducking their heads under the low rafters. These were boys I'd known since we'd first moved to the house when Jimmy was fourteen, teenagers from the local state schools, grown into lanky young men whose limbs seemed too long for them, with lots of hair and deep voices who filled the kitchen and delighted the small children with their great size. Sometimes, on the days when the feeling of my sister's death had crumpled me completely, I'd see them, arriving at the house and walking to the barn with a look of pure intent, snapping lighters, skateboards under arms, their laughter the sound of camaraderie playing out, and I would feel in awe of them. Yes, awe. Watching from an upstairs bedroom as I stood up from my desk after writing for the afternoon, I was envious of their friendship, and also of the time they had, lying stretched out before them like a brilliant multicoloured rug, huge, expansive, waiting. The virus had screwed up their lives, their education, their plans, but they wore this disruption lightly.

One weekend in the summer they drove to Devon, and I watched their little convoy of three cars vanishing from the yard, music blazing into the summer afternoon. I thought of the way Evangeline asks me to put music on in the car. Often I do, but sometimes I say I can't because if I hear loud music I won't be able to think properly. I envied the way the boys had the music turned right up before they'd even left the yard, all their cars playing different kinds: one of them had techno, one was playing Eminem and one had reggae coming from it. I envied them the optimism of everything they did. I knew they were driving to a beach to make a fire and take drugs and I envied them. I wanted to be a teenage boy driving to the end of the country to take drugs for the weekend to shed themselves of everything, because mostly they were still too young for life to have broken small parts of them away. I cannot even listen to reggae any more. I have a small scar on the edge of my eye where my eyebrow was split open by a man who was in a reggae band and who I'd been seeing for a few months in my early thirties. He locked me in his flat and put a knife to my neck as he cut my face with a mirror and raped me while reggae played, and now every time I hear it, I think of that man and the fear I felt. I'm telling you this because writing about it takes the power from it. People say to me about my writing: How can you do this? How can you be this open? Don't you mind other people knowing so much about your life? Don't you have any shame? But I am

not ashamed of this. And writing about it, and all the difficult, painful things I've been through in my life, is exciting;
it's as close as I can come to the feeling those teenage boys
have as they drive away to take drugs and be free. It makes
me feel my skin is thin. But I must feel it all again, too, in
order to write it honestly for you, so I think that it might be
one of the most painful and true things I have brought upon
myself.

The boys had stopped using the barn as a skate park in the
summer, so after we brought the Shetlands home in Bill and
Sally's trailer, I disassembled the skate ramps made from
pieces of plywood and secured them around the edge of
the barn to create a stable for the ponies. A farmer brought
me several bales of hay and the ponies looked snug in their
new home. There was a light in the new stable so even
when it was dark by teatime I could be out in the barn, filling hay nets or buckets of water for the ponies.

   The Shetland ponies were shy at first, uncertain of the
way I moved around them in the stable. I bought tiny
halters from the horse-feed store near home, and some
small brushes and hoof picks so that in the evenings after
school Evangeline and Dolly would come out to the barn
and tend to the ponies. We used the brushes to comb the
knots out of their hair and the blacksmith came and cut
their hooves back so that the ponies looked more comfortable while the children were leading them around the
yard. Bill and Sally sometimes came over to the barn in the
evenings and we'd sit as dusk arrived, an orange glow from

the end of Bill's cigarette between us, and talk about horses some more, or death, or what Sally might cook Bill for supper.

I don't know if it was the ponies, or the travellers, or time itself, but sometimes I'd catch myself talking about my sister, and at the same moment realize that it didn't automatically make me feel sad. In the hours that I spent with Bill and Sally, sitting in the barn with the Shetlands while Evangeline filled their hay nets, or talking about horses, or making jokes about where to buy and maybe sell more horses, I sometimes told them about her. Neither of them had ever met her when she was alive, but since hers was a world of horses and wagons and canaries and greyhounds and golden ornamentation, they liked hearing about her. When I talked to them, I could exist in a golden light of the best stuff about her. I could conjure her up for them. She wasn't existing in my heart then, or as someone who was always part of me, which is where people had told me to look for her, but was a being separate from me but belonging to me, in the barn with us.

One evening in late September when it was dark by early evening, I found myself searching through a cookbook for a recipe she had told me about. It was for potatoes cooked slowly with cream and cardamom and a cinnamon stick. I found it in a recipe book with a missing cover and broken spine, one I'd given her for her birthday, the inscription in the front told me, when we went to see a show called *Saltimbanco* by Cirque du Soleil at the Royal Albert Hall.

The date in the book said it was 2003 and I remember I had been given press tickets since I was writing about the show. We met at High Street Kensington tube station and walked up to the Royal Albert Hall and I recall seeing a long line of people in black tie and jewel-coloured dresses queuing up in front of the box office and only then understanding that this was a big deal. My sister saw a golden woman wearing black who looked like Claudia Schiffer and then we realized it was Claudia Schiffer.

We had been given a box where we sat and drank Moscow mules because that was the only cocktail we both knew well, apart from martinis, but neither of us wanted a martini. Sometimes my sister leant over and whispered to me about having met one of the clowns before or that she'd seen that gymnast perform in another country. She knew everything about this circus, and many others, and I realized she could see inside the magic of it. Like looking at the ponies in the dark without staring right at them, she knew how to find things that were not always apparent in the mess of life. Afterwards we rang up our dad and told him about it. He laughed when we said, 'We had cocktails,' and he kept repeating it over and over. It made him happy.

Looking through the cookbook as I stood in my kitchen, I could recollect that evening very clearly and I also made a mental note of the fact that writing in books is a good thing, and even better is to add some kind of detail. If I hadn't written in that book that I'd given to my sister when we went to see *Saltimbanco*, there's absolutely no way I would have remembered that. But in one line of messy biro writing (I have really terrible handwriting) preserved on the inside of a cookbook, a whole moment and whole evening in my life with my sister fell into my lap.

It was a complicated recipe which demanded that I not curdle the cream. The first time I made it I failed to do this and ended up with a sort of eggy potato pudding absolutely no one wanted to eat so I had had to feed it to the chickens. Now I made it again while the children watched *The Sound of Music*. They have watched this film about ten times and never get bored by it. They especially like the sense of peril in the nerve-wracking ending and sometimes they just watch the ending on its own. I do not want to pass trauma on to my children, but I sometimes wonder if it's not inevitable?

Anyway, untraumatized, at least for now, they were watching the film as I slowly cooked the potatoes and cream, and that sweet, spiced smell of cardamom was all around in the kitchen. I was using a heavy red cast-iron pan my sister had given us when we got married. It made me think of the many times I had been in the kitchen with my sister as she was cooking something. She was a good cook and before the last few years of her life, when she didn't really seem to like cooking any more, she produced funny things like a chicken she had spatchcocked and cooked with tequila. She always made her tables look beautiful. Even when Jimmy and Dolly were small, and I'd turn up just for tea at her house on a Friday night (something we did a lot), she'd have laid the table with a cloth and put pieces of lemon cake and flapjack on a nice plate or even a cake stand. Even if the cake was just one she'd bought in the

Spar shop, when she put it on to a proper plate it somehow turned it into an occasion or even a celebration.

Maybe it was the calming effect of the slow-cooking potatoes and the sweetness of the cardamom, and the hypnotic way I had to keep staring at the cream and stirring so that it was just hot enough but not so hot it turned into chicken feed, along with the sense that the children were all calm and not about to flare up and start throwing plastic around, but I felt a deep and absolute sense of joy. It wasn't exactly a feeling that she was there, but it was a quiet sense of the rightness of things, which was very comfortable, especially in comparison to how wrong they had felt for so long. And even if I had curdled the cream, I still think the rightness would have been there. A solidity in the presence of life, which was the children, the cream, the cardamom and heavy red pan, and also a solidity in the presence of death, which was my sister and me, since we were somehow *both there*, and also *both absent*, in that moment in the kitchen.

I had stopped staring at the face of death and, in doing so, I was starting to see it more clearly. I was still under the spell of death, but I also knew, quite clearly, for the first time, that it was a spell which often felt like a dream. And perhaps it wouldn't go on forever. Dreams do end, after all, even as they stay with us.

Later that evening, the children were in bed and I was on my computer looking back through some old emails for a poem I had sent to a friend that I wanted to read again.

Quite suddenly, between hundreds of old emails I was scrolling through, a message from my sister appeared with the subject line: 'Cook this'. It was written on 8 December 2009 at 4.20 p.m., exactly a decade to the minute before she died. She wrote to me:

> this is the recipe I told you about i think cos its from memory so you could maybe try it this week it was totally yum when I made it
>
> smash up and fry onion, bay, garlic, chilli, a cinamon stick cardamon
>
> add chopped fresh tomatoes and fry up
>
> add peeled pot chunks
>
> add coconut milk and simmer cook the lot, the milk just covering the solids.
>
> YUM
>
> would love to have a proper gossip some time soon.
>
> Love you.

Distraction is the best way that I can describe the state I went into during the autumn. Having four Shetland ponies in the barn was distracting. The ponies needed me, and crucially they needed me outside the house. They didn't need me in the way the children did. It's hard to nurture the lives of young children when you are pressed up against death and when you have been in the room with death and sat near it while it takes your infinitely precious pearl away with it. Because at the same time that I was riding with Galahad and Gawain into some of the most frightening territory of my life and trying to fashion some meaning or explanation from it, I also needed to be a mother. But when I was outside in the barn with the ponies, there was an elemental clarity to the way I was existing. Filling up buckets of water or mixing a feed, even mucking out, is calming. Walking around in the outdoor world is intensely soothing. The Shetlands just gave me a reason to do it.

Evangeline and Dolly were part of the pony project, and sometimes I could persuade Dash and Lester to be part of it too. Evangeline liked to tie all four Shetlands up in a row, giving them a tiny scoop of pony mix each, then taking the little brushes and smoothing the knots out of their manes. One of them was wilder and tougher than the others and didn't like being caught or led around, but the little grey that Evangeline called Pegasus and the skewbald named Minnie, and the chestnut who didn't seem to have a name, would nestle their muzzles into the crook of our arms as we stood by them. They resisted a little to start with but then they seemed to like being led around the yard and up and down the road towards the green.

There was something about the size of the ponies that was manageable too. They were almost small enough to pick up. They did not ask for much and didn't need shoes or expensive feed. They were easy to be around, and that made me easier to be around, and my pain easier to be around because dazzling life was there.

Feeling a sense of rightness growing slowly around me over the course of that autumn was extraordinary. There were even days of joy. But although joy was there like small bubbles in my tea, I was still quite conscious of the fact that the altered place that death had taken me to, where I felt solitary and other, was still, perplexingly, the place I felt most at home. A sense of perilous unease existed all around those bubbles of pure joy, which was both a strange, sharp anxiety about where the feelings I had might be about to take me, and a sense of the sadness that must be borne through the rest of life. If I thought of the things my sister would not get to do, and the places she would not visit, and times she would not be there for, I felt broken in half. When I imagined those things I still felt as if I would fall to my knees. I still, often, had to walk out of the room if a thought suddenly winded me, just at the moment that Evangeline was talking to me about her gymnastics exam. I still couldn't bear the thought of years and years of life without her.

We were standing on a beach the summer before she died, having had crab sandwiches with our children, when we had very briefly tried to talk about death, and she had said to me: 'I cannot talk about it. I cannot talk about the pain of not being there to see my children grow up. I cannot bear the thought of not being with them. I cannot talk about the pain of not seeing you surrounded by your grown-up children. I cannot bear these things.'

When I thought about those words I started shaking inside and maybe that was part of my process of learning to bear them.

*

Bearing them was also about creating a new, different space around these feelings and the realizations they brought with them. Since I had identified that a place of presence and joy could be reached, and that for me it was outdoors, with the Shetlands and Bill and Sally – something I'd thought completely impossible at the start of the year – I wanted to work out ways that I could hold on to it and even fashion or wrestle it into regular moments in my life. I had had to give up smoking as tending to that little addiction wasn't really tending to myself. It was just tending to the nicotine addiction which I was mistaking as the feeling of missing my sister.

Many days of the year until then had felt like a challenge. First of all, my quest challenge had simply been to get up and walk through the days, rather than allow my sister's death to floor me. That was all I had needed to do in the very earliest days. I'd needed Galahad and Gawain and Lancelot with me at all times. While I'd definitely wanted to get on to their horses with them and ride two up (as I had with Dagir, through the high peaks of the Caucasus Mountains), I had also been aware that it was a mission I could only take up alone. Remember: ride into the darkest part of the forest alone where the frost is undisturbed.

But there were other things that I started consciously telling myself. Use the messages of life that Jimmy and his boys show you as they walk through the house laughing before they drive, still laughing, into the light; listen to the wisdom of others who have walked into the fire of the furnace. Look for the people and things who show you a new way. Find people who have walked this way before and study them. Be alert to the messages you see around you, which might take any form, even recipes. And walk into the face of the pain that's before you like Gawain: he did not resist the Green Knight's challenge. He bowed his head down before the green axe, revealing his white skin at the most vulnerable part of his neck.

By moving into the darkest part of the forest again and again as I faced my sister's loss and by learning to live with death alongside me, I was trying to force myself to stare into the most terrifying, and even grotesque, parts of existence. I was trying to look right at the feeling of what the end of existence, the end of a life, really meant.

By visualizing the path through the year as a quest, I'd created a safe place to exist with my memories. When language failed me, the image of the quest knight was there. Lancelot and Gawain had pulled me out of the place of confusion I was in, forced a sword into my hand, held a shield to my breast, and sent me into the darkness. They knew I could do it. They had done it. They were knights but they were also human and knew what a human could withstand in terms of pain. They hadn't sent me out to do something I couldn't do. They knew they could teach me what was bearable.

My sense of these myths surrounding me was not completely rational. I don't actually know a knight called Lancelot. Galahad did not actually ride down the King's Road with me (oh, I wish he had though♥!). But they were part of visual rituals which helped me keep walking in that year, since, when death pressed down all around as I stood in the corridor of Gloucester Hospital and took my sister away with it, just walking was a challenge. At that precise moment, I was summoned for a quest. And if I had not answered the call, if I had not ridden into it with all the armour the knights could press on me, there might have been a sense of another life lost. Not just my sister's. But my own, too.

You know that feeling, when you have depression, and you don't actually know you have depression, and so you don't know why the dislocated sense of distance and loss keeps bearing down on you, or what to do to manage it, let alone how to stop it? If you know that feeling (who doesn't? Truly? Is there truly any human life without pain?), then you will know how much clearer the route out of depression can be when you realize it's something you can actually name, rather than a terribly overwhelming feeling you do not understand. But when you understand that this is actual DEPRESSION and not just, oh, feeling a bit down, that's the moment when you can start actively doing something about it. Even if all that means is existing in the knowledge you have depression and knowing one day you will be able to stand up against it.

Nothing is more annoying though, when you are depressed, than being told that going for a walk, doing some breathing (duh!) and getting enough, but not too much, sleep is the thing that will haul you out of the seething pit of darkness. I was told by people during this year after my sister had died that I needed to find her in my heart, or do the things she had loved, or know she was always with me every time I saw a remarkable robin/star/butterfly. When I think of this now, I understand why it was always really annoying and never helped at all.

I had hated cooking the things that my sister liked since they just made me remember I'd never eat them with her again; it hurt going to the places she had loved as they made me step straight back into the vortex of pain; I was sick of butterflies; and I'd ransacked my heart looking for her but I didn't actually find her there. I was still alone after I'd ripped my heart open. But when I stopped doing those things, there she was.

How I saw myself, in what was now late autumn, was a bit like that moment I have just described to you when you realize you have depression. When I thought about much of the year, I knew, absolutely, I had not had depression, but I had most certainly been existing in a very altered state. In the autumn, one season from a year since death had pressed down and taken my sister, I was able to look backwards and see the past more clearly: it was like that moment I have mentioned of realizing depression is there. The realization itself is a relief since it liberates you from the feeling that you are going mad, or that your life is over. No, you simply have depression. An altered state of consciousness. This is why the moment with the potatoes and cardamom was so important. It was the time in the year when I realized I could be happy, and that happiness and presence and even optimism was something I could create.

I could be all those things and create them too, despite the fact that my sister was dead. Maybe I could create even more of those good feelings because of the death of my sister, not despite that fact. Death could show me how to live more absolutely, just as my quest with the knights was doing. And I had a quiet secret sense that my sister would do them too.

But I wasn't completely sure if this secret was true. I'd glimpsed it but it might have been a trick. So I didn't trust in it. Not yet.

Chapter 8

Various Kingdoms

In November, when Pete was still away in America and I was spending a great deal of time alone with the ponies and the children, a woman came to see me. She messaged me to say she wanted to talk to me about life and death. I had met her on Instagram and at first we had exchanged DMs, and then sometimes longer messages or emojis. I sometimes sent her a poem, and she sent me pictures of paintings. Her son had been killed in an accident about a year before my sister died. He was seventeen and had been electrocuted by a cable lying in a pool of water where he was working in a food-storage warehouse. Sometimes she posted pictures of him on her stories: a tall boy with very blond hair, a lopsided grin, slightly hunched as if he was trying to hide his height, half turning towards the camera. He was her only child.

Sometimes I looked at his picture when I was holding

my phone close to me at night looking for my sister, and I tried to understand where this boy, this woman's *only* son, might be too. He was like Jimmy, or one of Jimmy's friends, those optimistic boys driving into the horizon. I wanted to scoop back into the past and take him to his mother. Lift the wet cable out of the puddle, turn off the tap that had caused the flood, change time, change motion. Stop death in its tracks and put a bit more time and life around this optimistic, white-blond boy who was now dead.

I read about him on her Instagram feed and I started to look forward to her posts about him. In the little bright squares of light, he came alive for moments of time. Like the film clips of my sister, there was an immediacy to the slightly wonky video-camera angles and there was an intimacy to the way he was right there, in my phone which I clutched so tightly to me so much of the time, often lying in bed late at night, scrolling through images and always returning to this son and to my sister.

Soon after we started messaging, the woman and I knew we wanted to meet. We recognized a certain outline in one another we wanted to touch. We had had a plan to meet in London, but the virus was making things uncertain. Not entirely locked down, but not much movement either.

Since I could not meet with this new friend death had brought to me in a London cafe, she drove to my house, arriving at 10 a.m. She sat down at the kitchen table and we talked until 3 p.m. without ceasing, at which point I had to pick the children up from school.

Talking via our DMs on Instagram had given me a sense

that I knew her in some way, or at least knew her path, the way she was walking, the armour she was wearing. She too was a knight. She was very familiar and from the moment she sat down until the moment she got up to leave I felt easy with her, as if I could just reach out and take her warm hand if I was falling. Talking to her was as if we plunged into the same dark water and were swimming around with our breath held, trying not to let a fear of the underwater world overwhelm us, and sometimes reaching out and touching the very tips of each other's outstretched fingers.

She told me everything about the death of her son: the noise she had made when she heard what had happened; the way a friend had driven her to Lincolnshire where he was working; and that although she knew emergency services were with him there was no answer from his boss who had called her about the accident, 'and in those moments, I knew. There was no news, and so I knew.' She told me about sitting with his body after he had died, and wondering and wondering how she could communicate to him that he could leave her, he could go, but that she would follow, she would always, always be following.

'He was my only son, my only child, and I knew him like he was a part of me,' she told me, and tears ran quickly down her pale face, very simply and normally, like raindrops running down a pane of glass, and I was on the outside looking deep into her.

I asked her about her son: What was he like? What did he enjoy? What made him happiest? How was he as a boy? And as she talked about him the tears stopped running down her face but instead it was as if he was there, in the words she was telling me, in her memories, in the pure light of her love for him. I didn't know this boy although I had looked at his photographs a lot, as I told you, and in her same pale white-blonde hair, in the intonation of her voice, I could see him. Her bravery, too, enacted him for me.

While we were talking, I was aware of something I had thought about a lot in the last year, but also a lot since Mum's accident really. My friend asked about my sister, but she had lost her son. Her only child, who was just stepping into life. Her pearl. I respected her grief and the eighteen months she had walked through as something bigger, more powerful, a more intense furnace than mine. I was aware as we talked about it that the forests she had ridden through were darker, harsher, more clogged with brambles and wild animals than mine had been. She had lost her *only child*. At times, while she was sitting in my kitchen, talking, I was aware of studying her face and looking for clues about survival and resilience in her countenance. And I thought about fragments of memory I could recall in words from T. S. Eliot about the hollow men who look into death's various kingdoms but who are always alone. I thought about the way, in the past year, I had spent perhaps as little time alone as I ever had, since we had all been at home so much, but that my closer proximity to death than anyone else in the house had made me *feel* very alone. And that helped me understand something about the hierarchy of grief. This woman had walked absolutely alone through the forest as she bore the loss of her only child. The closer the

person we lose, the more lonely that path may be, and
there can be no closer loss than an adolescent child. The
child fully formed, but sheering off from you, seeing himself as separate from you. Hers was the ultimate loss.

Later, at dusk and while the children were shouting in the
kitchen, I went into the sitting room, which was cold, to send
this woman a message. When I looked up from my phone, I
realized I was looking at fairy lights I had hung the previous
Christmas in the sitting room but never got around to taking
down and some of them seemed to sparkle brighter than
other ones. I had not met this lady with her pale skin and pale
hair until a few hours before, but in some ways I felt as if I
was standing, if not right beside her, then at least very, very
close to her. When I was in her presence, I didn't feel alone
at all, but filled up with something else, something intan-
gible. I saw my heart for a moment as a small bright light that
had lit up beside hers. So many people had said to me after
my sister had died: 'I cannot begin to imagine your loss.' And
those words had sent me out alone into the year, into the
darkest part of the forest where the frost is undisturbed. But as
I walked on through the year, I saw I wasn't alone.

I wasn't alone.

More than anything, I wanted to communicate to this
woman: *I feel something of what you're feeling. I walk close
to you. My light is shining close to you. My light is shining
here for you.* And then I was confused, too, as I wasn't sure
if it was my light shining close to her, or that the light of my
sister had illuminated itself, close to the bright burning light

of her son. I wasn't sure which light I was truly looking at, but I knew that somehow, within the darkness and colour of death, we were standing together, united by a brighter sense of each another's humanity.

Being in the presence of this woman who had suffered such a great loss made me feel reassured and in a way more stable. Less bewildered, somehow, about how random and appalling life is. It's all random and appalling. It's all beautiful and extraordinary. All these things exist together all the time. Often, often, often I have looked around at other people with lives that didn't seem marked by profound loss and felt envious of them – quite often green with jealousy. There were the friends with mothers and sisters who were all alive and walking about on the earth, completely normal. A state of normal had been disturbed for me at sixteen. What happened to Mum altered everything, smashing big parts of my life; I have put these back together and made something new of them which is infinitely precious, as precious as the pieces that went before, but three decades later I know there are hairline fractures that run through everything inside me. Sometimes I feel that if I or life apply too much pressure, large pieces of me will break again. At other times I feel stronger, more stable, as if my life has been a process of stress-testing these fractures, and that perhaps I willingly put myself into certain situations because I knew those exact situations would apply the maximum pressure to the places where I was weakest. And there was something motivating in knowing I had survived a great deal of loss. Loss had kept me moving and made me do things. Loss and trauma had hurt a lot but had also been a creative force. I had wanted to know that I was as strong as could be, but since my sister had died I had felt that the cracks were deeper. I knew I could be as strong as cast iron, but, like cast iron, I could shatter too.

Maybe it was thinking or talking about my sister so intently with the woman whose son had died, but later, in a place I cannot clearly recall, I was aware of my sister being with me. Suddenly I was in the kitchen at home, and the kitchen was quiet and empty so perhaps it was early morning or late night. I remember thinking I was there, I must have been there, since our orange cats were jumping from table to chair, mewing at me, and the clock that belonged to my grandmother which I often forget to wind was actually ticking so I must have wound it up recently. I was in the kitchen and my sister was there.

It's OK, Clo. It's OK, Clo, it's all OK, it's OK, Clo.

Her hair was long and blonde, so I was seeing her as if she was a younger woman, before cancer. She was frowning a bit at me, that deep brow, as she often did, but also reassuring. *It's OK.*

Later, as I recalled this and tried to write it down, I realized my sense of what had actually happened and the space I had seen my sister in were confused. When I recall dreams they come from a deep place in my head, a bit like those ponies in the dark that I see more easily when I do not stare straight at them. But my recollection of my sister in the kitchen that time with her blonde hair around her shoulders was something I could stare straight at. I started to wonder if I might have woken up shortly after falling asleep and walked downstairs, more than half asleep, maybe worrying about a sound I'd heard, and imagined my sister was there, or mistaken Jimmy for her, then returned to bed without really waking properly. Or had I dreamed her? Maybe I'd actually seen her? I was so confused. Did I see her in a room in my house? Or feel her in a room in my head? I know she was there.

And later I realized: Does it matter? Does identifying the dimension in which I've been present with my sister make her more real? She was real to me in that dimension and isn't that everything?

The distraction I had been experiencing when I spent time outdoors, either with the ponies but also if I simply just stepped out into the cold autumn world, was a state that I found myself turning to more and more. I realized that earlier in the year I had wanted to press myself against death, since death was the place where my sister was. Close to death's petrol-blue beauty was a safer place to be than trying to be happy or even just feeling normal in my brightly painted kitchen, which was a big, jangled challenge that made my eyes flicker with the headache behind them. But there was another place I found when I was outside with the small, lively Shetland ponies, when my head would quieten and I would start moving through the landscape with something like joy. It was the opposite of the way I had moved through life at the start of the year, as if ill or poisoned. I realized too that I no longer needed to test her. I no longer needed to ask her questions and feel afraid of or angered at the silence that met me. I didn't need to desperately reach backwards to the time when she was alive because I started to feel, in glimpses, that she was the talisman at the centre of my life. She was there, at times, without me doing anything to force it.

One evening, I was in the yard outside the house with Evangeline. It was still and dry, the rain of the previous weeks having let up for a bit. It wasn't yet deep winter and there was still an autumn warmth. I could hear the chattering, busy noise blackbirds make before night. The farmer had dropped hay and straw off earlier that afternoon, so that one end of the barn was stuffed with the warmth of yellow, sweet-smelling bales. I had bought an electric kettle and a jar of instant coffee for me and hot chocolate powder for Evangeline and Dolly that we kept in the barn. My stepmother had given me a radio which Evangeline had tuned to Heart FM, so the barn had a sweet domestic feeling. Evangeline and I had been feeding the ponies, but as it got darker she peeled back inside to find Dolly, while I stayed out on my own, just a bit longer.

Being outside in the dusk with the blackbirds and ponies made me feel relaxed, and rather than go back into the kitchen I sat on the big stone trough beside the barn, resting the back of my head against the painted black boards of the barn, closing my eyes.

Everything left me, apart from the distant sound of the

birds, and, without wanting or willing it, behind my eyelids I was suddenly with my sister in the drive of the house I grew up in. She was present to me, and my mother was there too, just standing, happily and easily in the dim light, for it was dusk where they were too. It was an acutely relaxing feeling, and my body felt heavy, a sense of my being and my human form existing in all of me, right to my fingertips and toes. I knew my mother and sister were not dead because my father was there too, in the gathering darkness in the drive at and no one was saying anything, as there was no need to say anything. We were all simply present together.

The sense of being with them was so strong that I knew I did not need to test them, in the way I had unsettled myself testing my sister's presence by trying to talk to her and see her in signs. I opened my eyes and the yard at home, the last late evening light, the glow from the house, the ponies and their hay, were all still there, the blackbirds chattering. I closed my eyes again and I was back with my sister and my mother and my father. I opened my eyes and I was back in the yard at home. I closed them, and I was back with my mother and father and my sister. They were not close enough to touch but they were all there, although no real sound was coming from us, or from inside my eyelids, but I was aware of a faint rustle, like the blackbirds around me. And I could feel then that death and the indistinct but absolute shape it takes in the lives of the living was a kind of enchantment. It's difficult not to believe in the human spirit when you really consider our ability to withstand the loss that life brings with it. There's a magical alchemy to pain and life that we cannot explain and maybe a good life is not one that's easy but one in which we face a quest journey again and again. It is one in which we're called out into the realms of hard adventure and unknown new horizons more times than we think that we might be able to bear.

The moon had come out when I opened my eyes again. It was a crescent moon and although I could not see the entire shape of that blue globe, I knew it was all there, the darkness as well as the light.

Chapter 9

Three Black Horses

The path alongside death is crooked, remember. There are no consequential stages which happen one after the other, neatly, like dominoes falling. It's never as simple as that. When the clocks changed backwards and the year moved closer to the moment my sister had died, I remembered this. As December loomed, I did not think of the Christmas people had started to discuss but instead felt something tightening around my chest as if I was travelling towards the heart of all that this test had been about.

It was another shock and another reminder of how dark and confusing the forest could be. I walked the Shetland ponies around and around the yard, but I found it harder and harder to find that magical distraction they had been for me in the previous weeks. It got colder and sometimes there was frost in the grass when I walked out to feed them in the barn in the mornings. Before the children left for school, when I went back into the kitchen to make them breakfast, I would often walk around the kitchen, sprinkling cornflakes into bowls or wrapping little cheese sandwiches into pieces of greaseproof paper while actually feeling as if I was lying on the edge of a blade or a sharp knife. I felt as if I'd ridden through so much of the treacherous terrain with Galahad and suddenly I was falling again, failing again, stumbling as my sword fell from my hand, my shield clattering to the floor.

As December got closer, I could see my sister's death date looming bigger on my horizon. It was terrifying. It was a target I was moving towards and also trying to evade. When the children were not needing me I'd find myself back in iPhoto, looking at images of my sister and myself from six or seven years ago, before cancer was anywhere near our lives. I sometimes wanted to rap on my skull in the photograph and tell my future, younger self to look out, to *brace, brace.* I thought about the time I'd flown to Istanbul to see Pete, who was working there. I'd sat buckled up in my aeroplane seat and watched the cheery little safety video about what happens if there is a crash. The cartoon figures smiled at each other calmly as the woman took off her high-heeled shoes and the man prepared himself to slip out of the aeroplane on a kind of plastic slide.

Obviously, we know, don't we, that if we are caught in an aeroplane crash it's unlikely that the instruction to take off our stilettos first is actually going to save us. But in the video the passengers were all smiling as they went down the slide, probably to their deaths. I thought of my sister and myself as those passengers, sliding down to what might have been a kind of death for us both, although I saw that now I was moving beyond her, onwards, to something else without her. Not her birthday. Her deathday.

And as that day got closer I felt the knife I was lying on grow sharper and sharper. To stop it cutting me in half I had to make my breathing more and more shallow, so that its edges didn't slice me and leave blood dripping on the floor. It was extremely demanding, going about my normal life while at the same time my entire body lay on this knife. I knew it was requiring me to be brave, and I knew in those weeks just before the deathday that I was also taking my life extremely seriously.

One night I was on the sofa with Jimmy and Dolly, watching a documentary I had seen before about a Frenchman called Philippe Petit who performed an act of outrageous daring by walking on a wire between the Twin Towers of the World Trade Center. My sister and I had watched it about eight years before, and we had loved it. One of the reasons we'd especially liked it was because Philippe Petit looked strangely like our father when he was a younger man, and the funny thing was that my sister looked very, very like my father. So I felt as if I was watching a film with both my sister and my father in it as one person.

Outside the house it was very windy but there were logs crackling in the red enamel stove in the playroom. I felt safe and secure with my older children. Lying beside them, I felt protected by something bigger and more powerful than anything I was. It was their youth. With my younger children, I need to be able to protect them, to control them sometimes, to make their lives move in the right direction. This was a completely different sensation to the one I felt being with these young adults. I could be myself.

It was lovely to lie on the sofa with them and feel them on either side of me while the logs crackled, and in those moments I knew the petrol-blue presence of death was absent and there was nothing anywhere near us other than life. The burning logs were hot and I liked the feeling of slight confusion, or overlap, or life as a Venn diagram, which was happening to me, since if I let go of complete consciousness I wasn't absolutely sure if I was watching my dad on the screen, or my sister. Also, that the film was about a wire-walker was part of that melting sense of confusion, since wire-walking, circus acts, acts of human daring were all part of my sister's life.

Obviously to walk between the Twin Towers on a high wire is an immensely risky thing to do. It is also an immensely serious thing to do. Philippe Petit could not have done this in a casual way, or without thinking about it very, very hard. I could see that walking through the days of the previous year and back towards myself had taken all my concentration. It had needed me to take my life and my memories of my life with my sister extremely seriously. Walking close to death is a very solemn thing, but it's also something you are required to do while dealing with all the normal, stupid, dull and messy and funny days of your life.

I realized, lying beside the heat of the fire with my almost-grown-up children, that I was scared of those last steps, off the wire and back into my own life. It would take me further from her death, so that I worried my life and her death would no longer exist in the same Venn diagram. Walking close to death had given me an acute focus and now I was nearly back there I was afraid I might fail, just as I stepped off the wire.

I have never wanted to be involved in the circus. I wanted to be involved in my sister's life, but the circus was her world, not mine. I had spent a lot of time at her circus, but it wasn't my home at all.

People sometimes ask me about my involvement in the circus. They did so especially when my sister was not dead, when she was still alive. Quite often I was mistaken for her. We were physically similar, but she was much taller than I am.

'You have a circus!' a woman said, clutching at my arm expectantly when I met her at a lunch party in a garden in Wiltshire, maybe two years before my sister died. 'I have read about you, you and your travelling circus!'

She could have been one of many different men or women who have asked me this and I have always replied, 'No, I am the one without the circus, the one with all the children who writes about the way life feels.' Or words to that effect. I could see that this was a disappointment, but it didn't affect me at all.

'But you must be involved in the circus in some way?'

The woman in the Wiltshire garden stared at me intently, as if the very proximity of my sister's circus to my own life must mean I *had* to be involved in it. 'Do you perform?' She had cocked her head eagerly on one side as if she could will me out of what she must have felt was the mundanity of motherhood, journalism and writing and into a world which she (mistakenly) imagined was all glamour and sequins.

'No,' I said to her, 'I don't perform, except on the page.' People had always wanted me to play a role in this part of my sister's life, but I could not have wanted it less.

My sister sometimes used to laugh about this: 'Come on, Clo, slip on a catsuit!'

I can't imagine anyone will say this to me again. *Slip on a catsuit!* All the stardust has gone out of it now anyway. There were other things we said to each other that no one will say to me again. We could say to each other **PURE NEW WOOL** or **WATERING CAN** and it was like a secret code to games we played when we were adolescents that no one else understood which would make the other one laugh. **PURE NEW WOOL** and **WATERING CAN** were some of the very last words I said to my sister as she was dying. I whispered them to her while I pressed my face to her chest, where she was hot, and she smiled deeply and I felt her hand tightening on mine. She could not speak then but it was our secret code, finding its way to her as she left me so that we both knew we were with each other absolutely and always.

No one will say these things again, which is why I

have put them in their own special fonts to give them their own special place in this book of many other words about my sister and how I have lived without her. *Slip on a catsuit, Clo!*

Since she died, it was a relief to escape those circus questions. It was a relief to leave the circus, too. I spent a lot of time with my sister there, but that was because I wanted to spend time with my sister. I was twenty-four and pregnant with Jimmy when she started the circus. He had been born in the final week of the first season. I had wrapped him in a tartan blanket and taken him to the last show and felt as proud as a person can possibly feel. My sister had lived the circus with every atom of her being: she was an artist and a sawdust ring full of performing people was the vehicle for her art. You cannot imitate that. And that was a very personal thing because the circus also consumed her. Sometimes it was difficult to get to her through the layers of circus that surrounded her, even when I felt as if she wanted to reach out. But it made her feel safe too. The circus was where she could feel invisible.

'When I am in the show, I am no longer myself. That's a relief. No one can see me,' she told me one afternoon about four months before she died. The circus season was in full swing and we were on Marlborough Common, surrounded by wagons and performers. We had walked out on to the common. My sister's short white-blonde hair was covered by a long blonde wig. Her floor-length burgundy dress touched the dry, yellowed grass – it was mid-August – and she wore full, heavy make-up, black lidded eyes, red lips, diamanté clips in her hair, bracelets around her wrist, sparkling everywhere. We were talking about our mum and what had happened to her and to us all. My sister told me about a friend of hers whose father had fallen off a cliff on a family walk. She had said this friend and her three sisters felt as if they were forever trying to work out what just happened? What just happened? Their father's sudden death at that point in their late childhood had left them in a state of high alert. My sister was comparing them to us. We were always trying to figure out what had happened to Mum. And we talked for a few moments about how this affected all of us in difficult and complicated ways – my whole family, I mean – and my sister said she felt that too much had happened to ever really understand it or how it had changed us all since then, and that this meant we could not really talk about it at all, let alone honestly, any more. 'Too much pain and loss to go back into it now, to go back into what happened afterwards. Too big a can of worms,' my sister said, speaking in uncharacteristic cliché.

'I often feel I hate the circus. The demands of it. The endless people. It's horrendous. But it makes me invisible,' she went on, brushing the long hairs of her blonde wig from her top lip. Her burgundy skirts were stiff, moving around her in a full circle, falling beneath her corseted waist and for a moment I wondered how well we can ever know another person. She suddenly said, 'I'd really like to be a health and safety officer. Or work in a small giftshop in a small town and not have to do all this.' Then she looked at me very closely. 'Or I'd like to be back in the past with you and Mum.'

I had looked for my sister in places I thought I might find her, but after she died, she was completely absent to me in the one place where people imagined she would be: the circus. She was a work of art, even or especially in her death, and she took her art with her, like magic. Gone. Just sawdust and old curtains left behind. I felt relieved for her. She was invisible.

And now as I moved towards her deathday I could see how the circus was, without her, something entirely sepa-rate to my sister. It was just a show, slightly tarnished, and while I could see this happening, I could also see that can-cer was separating itself from her too. I felt as if I was walking back towards her and she was walking towards me, free from everything that had hurt.

And if distraction in the form of Shetland ponies and the outside world had carried me through the final season before her deathday, wonder moved me into the moment where I touched a year.

It was Tuesday and mist covered the landscape outside our house. Visibility was just a few yards. Life beyond my immediate vision was obscured. Normally I can stand at my front door and look towards the ancient and enduring line that the Ridgeway tracks on the horizon. At times when I have felt life moving beyond me, out of reach, it's reassuring. I look up at the Ridgeway and I know I'm looking at the exact position of an ancient track where women and men have walked and talked and prayed, cooked, fought, laughed, despaired, loved, fucked, cried, fallen, for thousands and thousands of years. That thought alone is consoling when the present moment seems to overwhelm me, or indeed, if the present moment just seems so insignificant I'm not sure what to do with it. Looking to the ancient past or the surreal future is sometimes helpful to remind me that these experiences have been shared by millions and millions of people around me, across time, like strings and strings and strings of little paper people all connected together, fragile and perfect, all completely unique and themselves but also all the same.

So I fixed my eyes on the horizon after I had thrust my feet into boots, pulling on my sister's red and black lumberjack coat (remember that one? *Does it matter if I look like a Canadian? That I might be going to chop wood?*), finding a pair of gloves and a three-quarters-eaten packet of fruit pastilles in one pocket which were all stuck together like a hard but sticky little stone. I needed to look at the ponies and to fill up their water buckets, drop some slices of hay into their hay net, but also to fill myself with the early-morning sense of the day and to try to breathe in some of its goodness to take away the anxious badness that can sit in my head in the mornings.

I think it was the first morning it had been really cold since autumn had started. It had rained a lot. There was sticky mud to slide through when I walked out into the field, so that I had had to keep the Shetland ponies shut into one stable and find new paddock space to rent down the village green too. The air had felt too warm and too wet through much of the previous weeks, hanging around as if in anticipation of something approaching, although when I thought more about it I realized maybe that was just me. I was hanging around in anticipation, unable to clear myself like mist. Instead, I fixed my eyes on to the horizon, remembering firmly that that's something we're often told to do. Stop looking down at your feet in the mud trudging onwards to nowhere and look up, to the light and the far horizon instead.

I had walked through eleven and a half months since my sister had died – which was close to 351 days – and occasionally, I could see myself like a mother, willing a baby who is just learning to walk, stumbling and falling and falling again, into taking her first steps and then walking alone. When I took my mind back to the weeks and earliest months after my sister's death, I could see that I had been almost as vulnerable as a very young baby, a newborn even. Her death had taken away our lives together as sisters, our childhood and adolescence and young adulthood, our history and relationship with one another, the memories, love, toys, fights, ideas, trauma, jokes, goodness, everything that we had shared, and so there had been a sense of my own death in life, too. The person I had been to my sister had died with her. That part of my person was gone. **PURE NEW WOOL** would always now just be pure new wool.

And in order to survive that death of mine – and, better, to exist and even thrive with it – I had had to learn to live again in this new, changed, completely different world, without my sister in it, like a newborn baby must learn to live. I had had to learn to walk again, and walk upright, not hunched and braced, shuffling around unable to face life, as I had so often found myself walking in the first few weeks after my sister had died. I had had to learn to feel life and see the goodness of it, the brightness of it, the brilliance and colour of it, even when blackness and despair had so often covered my eyes. And now as I walked towards her deathday, I could also see myself, a mother, arms outstretched, nodding at that toddling baby, smiling, reassuring, saying, 'You can do it. You can walk. Don't worry when you fall, you can do it, you can walk. And one day you will run.'

In the barn the ponies' breath was warm as I splashed water into their buckets, reaching out to touch and feel the golden warmth of their hay. In between thinking about babies and death as I went through these tasks, I thought about Galahad. Walking close to death after someone you love has died often feels like an experience beyond words, which is why the images of Galahad and Gawain had helped me. The vivid, ritualized images of these myths had helped me find my way, simply into and out of days, when I had wanted to give up and vanish into nothing.

Since the anniversary was approaching, I was worried that I should have something to show for the journey I had taken, because just getting through those days had been hard. A talisman of some sort – a personal grail, if you like. I needed something to hold out to the invisible knight spurring me along that said to him: *This is the lesson you have taught me and these are the things I have learned.* I kept feeling as if I only had to walk a little further and I'd find whatever it was that Galahad had sent me out to quest for. I'd find the thing I was looking for, and I'd find something that had been lost.

But in my hands I had nothing. I could find nothing to hold on to from this time, nothing substantial, I thought, grasping at the bale of hay as I threw parts of it to the ponies, feeling its elemental golden grassy goodness in my fingers. I remembered the way people had expressed their sympathy for my loss, and how I had wanted to run through our home looking for my sister. But she was simply moving, fast, to a place further and further in the past. The virus had accentuated that massively too. I was now living on a completely different planet to the one that she knew. I have experienced this sense before, as our mother had had her accident before mobile phones even existed and certainly before the internet was part of our lives. Sometimes, my sister and I would talk about how Mum might have navigated the world of computers and screen time and Google. We didn't think she'd have liked it that much, and it made the separation we both felt from our mother, and the division between our world as young adolescents in which Mum had been present, and our world with her after the accident, more acute.

And now that sense of separation between different worlds felt more and more intense. In lockdown I knew I spent hours and hours on my phone every day. Your average daily screen time last week was 9 hours 28 minutes, my phone would tell me. When that happened I'd close my eyes quickly and put the phone face down, reassuring myself that Dash had possibly spent nine hours on my phone at the weekend alone. He pushed my average up. But I could not permanently lie to myself and get away with it. I worried that each month or year I moved away from the time that my sister was here, I was becoming more digital. One day, probably quite soon, I would have an app on my phone to tell me when I'm infected with a virus, and a microchip in my brain to turn the heating on when I'm cold and crying and missing her. I thought of her as lucky. She would from now on always be ancient and mystical, while I was becoming dystopian.

I was thinking a lot about her deathday as I walked back to the house, bracing myself for domestic life, when three midnight-black horses walked out of the mist and through the gate into the yard. Every inch of them was black, from their tautly tangled manes to their strong black hooves, which were unshod, no glint of metal there. One of them was the size of a small horse, with a broad chest and high back, and a long mane almost to his shoulder. He looked like a horse you might ride into battle on. He was followed by two slightly smaller ponies, broad but not so tall, strong in their legs, footsure, the kind I scroll through equine websites for, searching for the right safe, brave, excellent animals for my children to learn to ride on. The three of them all turned to look at me as I stood silently in the yard, their coal-black faces watching me, their breath coming in plumes from their soft, velvet noses and heating the misty white air. Slowly, they picked their way across the yard, their metal-less hooves making no sound on the concrete.

I was holding my breath.

I felt as if I had been searching and searching and searching and when I had stopped searching the world had delivered. Unshod and unbridled, these animals were a concentration of pure black horse which felt like magic appearing through the mist at a moment I needed to be told that the world is beyond our understanding of what miracles and magic really are.

The horses moved gently around the yard and then towards me. Their movements were beyond words and beyond the stillness of the mist and the air enveloping me and everything I felt; all the hurt and the sadness and life lost was held around me by the mist and the ponies were present to it too. The ponies were present to the morning and present to me and present to the strange, still pain and the extraordinary human beauty of being alive on that morning. There was only that moment as they strained their necks to reach out their velvet noses, moving closer and closer and closer to my human touch. Their blackness was extraordinary, no tiny glimmer of white was present on any part of them, and that blackness made the green of the late-autumn grass, still so glistening and alive even as winter arrived, look even brighter and more brilliant under their black hooves. To be in their presence felt like the most profound and strange gift on that otherwise stone-cold normal late November morning. There were rewards waiting after pain. Galahad and Gawain did not return from their quests unharmed. Soldiers did not come back from battle without wounds, which mark their hearts as much as their bodies.

The black horses stood before me, breathing and watching, all still and quiet, as though they were everything in the world and also all the world, waiting for me. And as the biggest pony's muzzle brushed the tips of my fingers, acknowledging our breath and our hands and our sense of existing as live beings beside one another, I was aware of a thought. It darted through the sideline of my vision, in that fast, darting way a blackbird moves through the air when it flies to its nest at dusk, and this thought told me that I was wrong to think that the path I had walked had not been without change: death had forced me to remember that the world, and all its magical salves, was still waiting, quiet, healing and patient, as I walked back towards it. Distraction had propelled me across the previous few months as I sought my place outside, in the yard, in the barn, in the fields, but I now could see that death had revealed life to me as a place of wonder, in all its light as well as its darkness.

Of course you could just say they were ponies from a neighbouring farm. Winter was almost upon us and grazing was getting scarce, so they had broken through an insecure wire fence and walked down the road before wandering into our yard, since the gate was open. And it's true; a girl arrived a little later, clutching a red head collar, laughing about the ponies, apologizing for them having found their way to me, words tumbling from her mouth, a messy pony-tail of damp hair glistening with drops of mist escaping from an elastic band. She told me they were Dale ponies, bred for their courage and strength, and there was a complicated story she explained twice about the fact the ponies normally lived in Scotland, where she was a shepherdess, but she'd come south to have a baby, although she really wanted to go back to Scotland as she missed the hills and her life there.

She kept saying she was so sorry they had disturbed me, and I said again and again that it was no problem for me, that I loved her ponies walking into my yard. I didn't say what I was really feeling, which is that I wanted to thank her for her ponies disturbing me, since I had wanted to be disturbed. I had wanted to be woken up. Because death and life had walked into the yard that morning and I knew at that moment that it was something of what my quest across the year had been about. To see there was nothing wrong with pain. The blackness of the ponies was the wonder and mystery of a kind of pain. And if the past year had taught me anything, it was to live through all the outer edges of my life, even the bits that hurt so much, and not just say that I'd been there for the number of days of it. Death had shattered the globe of my life, and in order to survive that shattering I had put it back together even as it cut me open so that I could see all sides of it. Blood was everywhere, all over the floor, and although I did not know why it was so red, I was no longer afraid of the brightness of it.

My sister's deathday was only a few days away and I thought about it all the time. If it had been her birthday we might have been planning a party: coloured cakes and golden champagne with tiny bubbles poured into flutes. Actually, my sister did not like her birthday at all. Sometimes she planned parties, but she usually cancelled them. Once a close friend of hers took her to a very expensive Japanese restaurant with two other friends. My sister told me about the evening, laughing away how perplexed she had felt by it, because the music in the restaurant was so loud she said it was like being in an underground nightclub. She was in my kitchen, snorting into her cup of tea when she told me: 'Like being in an actual rave and eating seaweed while trying to have conversation at the same time.'

Lots of these kinds of conversations I'd had with my sister were now sitting in my brain like little clouds as her death-day got closer and my breathing got shallower. I thought of how we had celebrated her birthday, three years before, in early January, when we had ridden along the Ridgeway close to my house on two dapple-grey ponies she had bought when they were very young, and how afterwards we had both said it was one of the best days of our lives.

The virus we were all still living with meant that a large gathering of people or a party inside a house wasn't possible. Instead, I called a group of people who had mattered a very great deal to my sister and asked them to come to my garden. I could not let the day pass without something joyful happening. My sister's deathday had to be about joy as much as her birthday might have been.

My father and stepmother arrived earlier than anyone, since they'd been at the stonemason's organizing the head-stone for her grave. They had arrived with two bits of stone:

one with my sister's name carved on it; another with 'LAND OF MAGIC' and engravings of plants, like ivy, twisted around the words. These were not her actual stone, of course, but instead bits of stone that the mason had been practising on and that he had given to my father. My father opened the boot of his car and there they were. We lifted them out together, just as if we were lifting a very heavy suitcase out, and in that moment I was more proud of my father than perhaps I had ever been, both our hands clasped around the heavy edges of a daughter and a sister's grave-stone. My father wanted me to look at them very closely. He told me that the stonemason had said the chisel had moved in his hand as if by its own will and I thought again of the noise my father had made at the moment his daughter, my sister, had been dying.

'The way the chisel moved, and the lettering, the ivy carved around it, that's art,' my father said as we stood look-ing at the stones. 'She was art. She was always, always art.'

I felt nervous before the party, distracted as we laid out a long table which we decorated with golden chocolate coins and piles of bright orange tangerines and Quality Street sweets like pink, purple, yellow jewels scattered across the tablecloth. I bought ginger cake and small mince pies over which I sieved icing sugar, not so much to make it look as if I'd made them myself, although there was that, but just to make them look more tasty, and I cooked two trays of sausages with mustard and honey on them and baked some cheeses. One of them I dropped as I took it from the oven, nervous now, my heart pounding, because we were all here for death and that clash of love and death disturbed me. The cheese spilled on the floor, yellow fat oozing, but I scooped it up and threw it into the bin and instead carried just one cheese out to the table. Pete had lit a fire and we moved the firepit – one of those ones that's portable – under the veranda that runs around two edges of our house. Dolly brought out candles in storm lanterns. I took that same big red saucepan I had cooked the carda-mom potatoes in and made mulled wine, oranges sliced in half and studded with cloves bobbing around in the liquid, remembering a Christmas when Jimmy and Dolly were quite small and I'd stayed with my sister. 'Shall we mull another one?' she'd said frequently and now I remembered the way she sloshed two whole bottles into the saucepan. I put a photograph of my sister out on the green-painted wooden table, surrounded by blue benches and a bright pink chair. The big plates of food, tangerines and walnuts and all those jewel-coloured sweets and gold chocolate coins scattered down the table looked magnificent.

I was propelling myself forward through the day and as my brother and sister-in-law arrived with their two sons, and then another cousin, and three friends, I felt as if I was there, but I was also disturbed. Part of me was worried my sister might actually turn up and see the pieces of gravestone, which were propped up on the edge of the veranda. I really worried they would make her think she was inside a night-mare, since how could looking at your own gravestone be anything but that, and she would not realize that the whole party was a celebration of her. It was a celebration of her life and her death and all the power of it: that was why we were there, for her, for her life and for her death.

I sat at the table beside the burning fire with my family and some of my closest friends, hearing their voices but also feeling as if my own voice was somewhere else, floating separate from the table. I could not eat any of the coloured sweets or the ginger cake, and when I looked for the hot cooked cheese it was all gone, eaten quickly by everyone, maybe because it was December and, because of the virus, we were outside. But that was also nice, the fresh clean coldness of it all. There was no way you could just sit there and drink too much of the mulled wine and feel sleepy. It was much colder and sharper than that. Since I could not really eat, or talk coherently either, I just sat quietly and watched the faces of the people I loved, and I tried to feel what the presence of death meant now.

I had wanted to feel wonder, as I had when the three black ponies walked into the yard, but despite the magnificent table, the perfect powdery sugar sieved on to ginger cake, and melted cheese, and clove-studded oranges, I didn't feel what I actually wanted to feel until later that night, after it was dark. My brother and father had had to leave, because it was Sunday night and there was a drive back to London to do, but I hadn't wanted them to go. They were leaving when it was nearly dark, just as I was starting to find the actual feeling I had hoped for. I felt as if the death-day party was suddenly over too quickly. We had pushed the long table away from the benches. The beautiful table was covered in stained glasses, empty cups with grains of coffee in them, some melted wax stuck to the tablecloth, splashes of wine, the rubbish of sweet wrappers. But still we were out there, in the night and the cold air. And then at about six, two of my sister's very, very best, closest friends arrived; Nancy and, moments later, Emma. Their voices made me feel as if my sister was arriving with them and maybe she was. I found some more pieces of wood to burn and stopped stacking dirty plates at the table and instead embraced these two women, pressing my cheeks into Nancy's and then Emma's face where I could feel wetness on their faces too, because the reason that brought us to the table and the fire was my sister, but it was also her death. We did not want that to be true although it was impossible to avoid it. Death and love at the table together, but perhaps easier to bear now in the darkness than it had been that afternoon, because the table was so messy: no need for things to look magnificent, but simply to be. The door into the kitchen opened as Dash and Evangeline ran outside to see Emma's children, taking them quickly and climbing over the fence from our garden into the boggy field beside it. Further across the field, in the dark, I could hear the children's voices moving away from the house to test the edges of the darkness, furthest from the fire, which was burning very brightly now, with the new logs there.

I had known I could not let my sister's deathday pass with only a sense of sorrow and loss, and sitting beside the fire with Emma and Nancy I could find the joy and awe I had wanted. There was a crackle on the fire from a huge bunch of rosemary Emma had brought with her from her garden.

'What shall we do with it?' we laughed, and because rosemary is for remembrance, I threw it into the fire. It made the fire burn even faster and hotter and the sound of Nancy's laugh was something that belonged to a time when my sister was there, since they were so often together. For a moment, it was as if my sister was with us, but now I was not scared she would be horrified. It was dark – she would not see the stone with her name on it, but instead just see the party and the crackling hot fire.

While we were sitting by the fire talking, a feeling came over me which was like the sensation that I'd experienced when I had been cooking the cardamom and cream in that heavy cast-iron saucepan. This feeling was that my sister and myself were both present and together in the act, and both absent. I cannot remember what I spoke to Emma and Nancy about, but I heard something in my voice, which was a sound of her. Not the sound I'd heard after she first died, when, as I told you, I felt my voice became much deeper, as if she was inside my voice box, which had disturbed me at the time. It was not like that. It was not the voice of shock and death which I had felt so strongly immediately after she had died. Instead, it was the actual tone of my sister's voice. I felt it, too, in a certain gesture I made, without thinking, while we were talking. This was the feeling I had been trying to locate all day: a closeness, an end to separation. And at that exact moment I was feeling my sister inside me, Emma said: 'In that way you move your hand, that gesture, you are just like her.'

So I knew I was not imagining it. I had felt it, but Emma

and Nancy could see it too. After that I was very happy although I said nothing. I was very happy because I felt as if my sister was there, inside me, and she could not be taken away from me as I could not lose something that was part of myself.

Just then I realized that a small miracle had happened and that I did have something to show for the last year. I had learned that the dead do accompany us, even though it wasn't something I could have seen straight away. I needed to walk through the jagged edges and most painful places of the past year in order to see the new shape of my relationship with my sister emerging. That shape would never be one that I wanted, and I would always want her back alive, but there was comfort, certainly, in knowing part of her would be with me for ever. I couldn't lose something that was inside me, and actually was me, since I knew she was there, as bright as the red of my blood.

The party for my sister was several days ahead of her death-day, and each moment that took me closer to that date of 8 December felt as if a brace was tightening around my chest and making my heart beat extremely fast. Simultaneously there was a persistent ringing in my ears because what I was thinking about more than anything was my sister's body. I couldn't stop myself worrying about it, buried so deep underground in her blue and gold star dress with the letters and photographs and small talismans we had put into her coffin with her. I wanted to know if her body still existed inside the world.

I kept having images in my mind, both when I was waking and asleep, of how her body would be, and this required me to do all I could to silence the alarm again in my head. I felt a little bit like I was bracing myself to do anything I could to resist the actual deathday arriving, but that because I couldn't, time was leaning on me, pushing me forward with all its might, just to get to the day, to feel it all around me, to stand inside the moment, a year before, when my sister had died.

Partly to stop myself spending any longer at my computer googling *How long does it take for a body to decompose*, and partly to allow my eyes to settle on a new landscape and be silent, away from the children, I drove south, into Wiltshire, to stay at a friend's empty house for two nights, alone. I needed to write down all these words for you. I needed to write all this down because I wanted to share with you the things that have happened in the time since my sister's death and the difficult, precious experiences I have lived through.

An empty house, alone with myself and the thoughts in my brain, without a dishwasher that needed emptying, school uniform that needed folding or Lego that might be trodden on, barefoot, seemed like the most serious place I could be to think back on what had been happening over the last year, and where I had arrived at in the forest.

To be in my small car alone driving across the downs, deeper into Wiltshire, was a new joy after the many different kinds of confinements of the previous twelve months. The sky and horizon seemed bigger and greener, the distances further, and even the cars on the grey road around me seemed faster than ever. I was flying in my car, suddenly flashing down the A303, and there was Stonehenge, those rocks like huge graves in the middle of this massive landscape, ancient and eternal, talismans and secrets, embodying the blazing glory of humanity's pain and hope. They were a comfort and a release.

The house I stayed in was empty but there were clean sheets on a double bed and clean towels by a shower. No oven, but two rings to heat up food that I didn't use, since for three days and two nights I ate nothing but some packets of cold smoked mackerel, sliced cucumber and tomato with sea salt, and oatcakes with either Marmite or peanut butter and jam. I didn't want to have to think about food. I just wanted to think about my sister and my knights and death. For two days I sat at the long table in the little house and wrote down many of the words you have been reading. Sometimes I stood up and walked around, or drank cups of instant coffee, and twice, when I couldn't concentrate, I went and lay on the double bed and made myself come. It was easier, now, to move between words and sex than it had been a year before and I no longer felt the guilt that had made me cry the first time I had had sex after my sister had died. And making myself feel something good made me think of desire, and the need to assert my own life over the death that I thought of so much of the time. When I wanted to escape thinking about death, being inside this feeling of sex gave me the opportunity to inhabit new spaces inside me.

On 7 December, the day before my sister's deathday, and the last day to a year that we ever spoke aloud to one another, since she was unconscious on the last day of her life, I found my heart pounding very fast and I had to lie in bed, making a conscious effort to breathe slowly, to make myself go to sleep.

The sky was the colour of a new bruise when I woke up on her day, and I went outside where I could hear blackbirds lighting the dawn with their bird voices. The air smelt good, of fresh new earth and coldness. All around me the birds' voices chattered, telling me that this was the very day, the very day, the very day she had died. But it wasn't in the morning she had died, it was at 4.20 p.m., so there were still hours I had to get through, like a test approaching, before the actual moment of death.

I had taken with me to the house some of the little collection of objects I mentioned to you which made me think of my sister – my beads, the metal head of Jesus, the wooden bear I squeezed to countenance the unbearable, a small but heavy brass hare which my mum had given my sister when she was fifteen – and I set these around my laptop as I worked. I also had a candle in a glass jar. It had been the candle burning beside my sister's bed as she died, and I'd kept it in my room at home although I wasn't sure why I had not been able to make myself burn it. I didn't want to just squander it on a normal day as there were perhaps three or four more hours' burning light left in it, but now I had it with me, and so I lit it. I sat writing with the candle and these small, important things around me.

I wrote all day, but my mind was continually occupied with trying to work out what I should do at 4.20 p.m., when the hour of her death arrived. I had to do something. A part of me felt as if I should be doing something solemn like listening to Gregorian chants or praying, and I knew my sister would have liked that, but when I looked up at 3.49 p.m., through the big glass windows that ran down one side of the house and out to the west, I saw that the sky was no longer a bruise but slashed open with bright light, so I went outside.

Crows rose from the beech trees all around the house as I paced across the field beyond, which was springy with moss. Just as I had been expecting to see my sister arriving at her deathday party a few days before, now I almost imagined I might see, over the crest of the hill behind me, Galahad and Gawain and Lancelot and Arthur returning to meet me. I looked out for their glinting armour and the glimmering, gleaming silk cloth of their tunics, their helmets studded with gems selected for the special occasion. I imagined them in the splintered sunlight having crossed steep and snaking paths through the darkest forest and having mastered a bleak terrain of snarling wolves and sharpest serpents. They would be holding a banner overhead to show that the battle – the quest – was over.

But they weren't there, just as my sister had not arrived at her party. Instead, the blackbirds darted between the black outlines of the beech trees. The knights, or my mental images of the knights, had been close to me through so many of the days of the previous year as I tried to navigate a new world without my sister in it that I was sure they would be waiting for me now. But I scanned and scanned the horizon and I couldn't see them and I couldn't feel them anywhere near me either.

The hour before dusk was the time of her death so perhaps that's why the sky became pink as the time moved forward after 4 p.m. towards the last twenty minutes that my sister was alive in the world. The sky glowed brighter and brighter as the outline of the trees grew blacker and the chatter of the blackbirds became more intense. I walked backwards and forwards between the trees, talking to my sister and to myself with a gathering calmness around me as time moved on because, as I walked, I breathed deeper and my heartbeat slowed a little, and a quiet realization and then certainty arrived that I could not conjure her up, or call up my knights either, and now I wasn't talking to her in the hope that she would answer. I wouldn't see her again, and I felt still, even as I walked, held for some brilliant time in the moment, aware, at last, that there would be no single moment when things made a new kind of sense. I could not expect my sister's death to provide anything so neat or obvious. There would just be time moving around me in one direction, which was ever forwards. The journey for me alongside her death would always be messy and the one truth I knew was that the path through and beyond the woods, which I'd walked for the last year, would keep snaking and twisting, and that there would always be times when the darkness of the thorn bushes cut out the light of the sun or obscured the bright greenness of the landscape around me. The sadness and darkness of the forest would forever be something I would have inside me, and I understood that the knights would no longer ride beside me, showing me the way forward, because now I was finding the path all for myself.

And as 4.20 p.m. moved towards me I remembered the feeling of the power of death pressing down in the hospital corridor, the unstoppable weight of it and the petrol-blue wings which were lighter now, so much lighter that they were just the blackbirds around me, darting into the dusk. I had to tell myself to breathe and breathe to take myself towards the moment and I didn't know what to do but to keep breathing. And 4.20 p.m. on 8 December arrived and the world kept turning around and around. I cried as I walked between the trees across the springy moss. At that moment I understood that my faith in the presence and existence of a human spirit is so strong *because* of our ability to survive and thrive after great loss and greater tragedy. We endure the unendurable when rational feeling says we should disintegrate. I remembered the voices of people who said to me, after my sister had died, *I cannot imagine your pain, I could not cope without my sister, you are so brave, I could not survive without my sister*, and I knew in that moment that the thing which had enabled me to live without her was a kind of alchemy of pain and life beyond my understanding or really anyone's understanding. That alchemy transformed the pain and darkness of loss into a newer, brighter life force which was what held my life together now, cracked and changed, certainly, but not broken beyond repair. And I knew in those moments, walking between the black lines of the beech trees as the sky shone bright pink, that the sorrow I'd carried over the last year might have been the biggest part of my life, and that understanding this had also helped me find strength in it, or grace, perhaps. That understanding had also taught me about trusting life, not freaking out in the face of what life had presented, but simply believing it. I could see, too, that I had not chosen to be brave as I walked through the year. I'd done it because I'd had to. And I also thought of that feeling of acute loss which had moved with me, so acute in the months after her death that it had made me fall to the ground, or gasp out. That sense of loss was changing shape, so that while I no longer expected my sister to appear to me, or be able to directly communicate with me, I also carried a newer kind of faith. Just as I know swallows will return each year, I am certain my sister will be present to me and will continue to love me, just as I love her.

I could see these things more brightly as I walked between the trees and the pink of the sky intensified but then passed so that it started diluting, a darkness spilling over it like inky water. My sister's death had forced me on to a quest journey, but it would not be the only journey. A good life might be one in which there is journey after journey. I knew that the darkness of the forest I had walked through would always call me back. *Come back. Remember how you made your way through here. Remember how sad you were. Remember how it had felt unbearable and see how you have borne it.*

And I know I will go back into the dark forest, and I will walk there again, but in the knowledge that now I know the way through, I will return into my own life stronger. The forest will remind me that I can be brave, too. If you could speak to Gawain (wouldn't we all love to talk to Gawain, who always sought wonder?) and you asked him which is better, the security of court or being out there, riding through the place where the frost was undisturbed, I am pretty certain he would say that the most important moment of his life would be when he left the security of Arthur's court and rode out to look for the Green Knight's castle. He might have been more secure in the court, but he was more alive out on his journey, and passing his quest was where he had become worthy as a knight, just as withstanding the pain of the loss of my sister had earned me a special kind of strength and resilience I hadn't known I was capable of.

Before I drove home the next day, I knew I had to go to my sister's grave. As I walked up the steep path to the graveyard on the hill above the churchyard, my feet slipped on the wet mud of the path. The rain fell heavily as I pulled the hood of my coat over my hair, raindrops resting in nettles, greenness around, because it was December, and winter had not yet taken on that hard blackness which arrives in January. Visitors had been to her grave, leaving her messages and pink roses twisted into the shape of a heart. The rosemary I had planted on the grave before was bushy and upright, and there was a red ribbon with a gold bell on it that one of my children had put there several months earlier. Her grave looked busier with these offerings, but the mound of soil had shrunk, as though the earth had breathed her in. New burial plots had joined hers in the graveyard, and I crouched down beside her bed, putting my hands on to the earth. Death had made me believe in life and the extraordinary power of normal people, the way we keep going, keep walking, until it's all over.

I thought of my sister's voice, laughing when we sat in that wild-flower field together. 'Death, I mean, it's probably quite a relief, a long sleep . . .' she'd said to me then, and I thought of these words now. Death, I had learned in the last year, is the invisible everything at the centre of all our lives. I was relieved, in a way, that I was learning to acquaint myself with it. Rain fell, drops settling around me, as I sat back on my heels. Although I knew this wasn't the end, I also knew that some kind of spell was over. Walking through a year to the day since I had last kissed my living, breathing sister had been the biggest and most important task I had ever completed. It was the most difficult thing I had ever done. There beside my sister's grave, I needed to talk to my father more than anyone else alive. I needed to hear his voice. The rain dripped from my hood down my face, but it wasn't cold as I crouched down on my heels and we talked.

His voice was completely beautiful for me to hear, and he was alive. His was the voice I have heard all my life and his was the voice I wanted to hear talking about Nell. We said how much we love Nell and how much we missed Nell. I told him about the treacherous forest I felt I had trav-elled through while I was looking for Nell, and the cold wet grass, and the frost that lay undisturbed where I had found my own path and how hard and lonely that path had been. I said that I felt I was leaving the path for now although I knew there'd be times I'd find myself back on it. I told him how I felt that Nell was moving further and further away from me, and also becoming me, and that the separation scared me less than it had. 'Is it that you feel death is nothing?' he asked me, and I stared at Nell's grave, the rosemary, the flowers, the rain falling, the nettles and barbed wire separating the graveyard from the field above it, and I thought of what death is and I shook my head.

'No, I mean that I think death is everything. I think death is everything.'

Afterwards, I left my sister Nell there and I also took my sister Nell with me as I walked back down the steep path to my car, through the trees, looking across the expanse of the valley. It was not that I had reached the end of the path, but the feeling of living close to petrol-blue death was over. I am living and walking close to life – closer, I now see, than I have ever walked before.

Epilogue

Some time after I finished writing down for you what these experiences of mine felt like, I read in a report that physicists in a laboratory in Chicago had found evidence of a fifth fundamental force of nature. At that time I had also been trying to read a book about the future of fossil fuels, and in this book I learned about the concept of deep time. It was described as one of geology's greatest gifts to the human mind, since it was something unimaginably greater than the timescale of a human life. There was a figure of about 4.5 billion years put on deep time, and I liked allowing my brain to float around on the concept of this in the certainty that my brain could never understand it. I thought of the scientists in the Chicago lab and how it might have felt for them to make a discovery which could rewrite human beings' current understanding of the universe. I had been so preoccupied by time and going backwards through it since Nell had died, but now deep time made me happy as I could see myself and Nell and all of us, every single one of us, like tiny, tiny, tiny fishes, shivers and flashes of silver, darting and diving around through a time so vast and magnificent that it was completely beyond any of our understanding.

And as more of this mysterious stuff called time passed onwards after the first anniversary of Nell's death, I relaxed a bit more. I was no longer grasping backwards; deep time and that fifth fundamental force of nature made me feel more free. Maybe Nell was all around me and she was one of the natural signs or animals I saw all about. Maybe she was that black cat which followed me sometimes when I was out in the fields, and which had such bright green eyes. But maybe that was just a black cat. I was no more certain about where death had taken her than I had been a year before, but I was clear that by journeying back into the past to find her, I had found my way straight to the present. I had learned, too, that my love for Nell was not finite. It was not limited or contained by the fact we were in the same room together, by the possibility we could meet in a cafe for lunch, by the reality of her life. Death had taken Nell, but the love we had shared meant something of her accompanied me onwards and would always be part of me, just as I would always be part of her.

And now I tell my children not to be afraid of the dark, too. Sometimes – often – Dash and Lester will pull me back to them, as they lie in their little beds, telling me they are afraid of the dark. And that makes me think of being a child in a bed beside Nell, and asking her to tell me when she shut her eyes, so that I would not be left, open-eyed, in the darkness of our room. I was afraid of what the darkness would reveal to me. Nell's death has made me stare right into the blackest darkness I can imagine and has sent me tumbling through deep time, reaching, grasping, clawing at some kind of certainty.

Now I understand that it's not possible to know, just as I will never understand the redness of my blood. Why is my blood so red? Why is it so red? I cannot know that, but I do know that as often as I need, I will tell this story, and that in looking for Nell, I found that the darkness might surround me, but that it no longer scares me.

Acknowledgements

Although my sister had had cancer for several years when she died, her death was so sudden that for quite a long time afterwards I felt as if she must have been killed in an accident. My family has experienced many accidents, and that shock and sense of apparently unendurable bewilderment that follows an accident was where I found myself after Nell died. I wasn't sure how to survive. The book I had been working on for a few months before her death fell away, since all I could now think about was death. I was in the trenches with grief, but I also knew the vivid feelings I was having were a special experience. I started to realize that I wanted to record how this infinitely valuable thing that death does, which is to consolidate all your love for and sense of shared life with the lost loved one in a terrifyingly intense way, truly felt. And Nell also asked me to write this book: 'Write a book about this' was one of the very last things she said to me.

Grief is often a solitary experience, and I have tried to be as accurate and truthful as possible about the way my sister's death made me feel, but I have made a conscious decision to write predominantly about my own experiences.

I have not written about my sister's beloved children, or any of her friends' feelings, for example, because their experiences of Nell's death belong to them and are not for me to interpret. I haven't written about my siblings and their feelings about the loss of our sister for the same reason.

I am indebted to Sarah Langford, for both her deep friendship and the numerous long conversations we have shared about death and life and all the good stuff. The notes I scribbled on the back of a broken CD case, a few months after Nell died, during a conversation I had with Sarah, locked in my car so that I could get away from my children, when I was first formulating my ideas about death, have become the book you are holding now.

Thank you, Rebecca Schiller, for your writing retreats, which are always a place for deep diving into stronger thoughts, and massive thanks to Helen Dyer for so much friendship, a whole lifetime of it, and for making me get out of bed and making me laugh (about yoga, of all things! I hate yoga!) when I just wanted to cry and die. Thank you, Gillian Stern, for always cheering me on and for your support for my writing over two decades. Deep thanks to Inigo Russell, who inspired me to think harder about Arthur and his knights, and who found the title of my book amongst my words, and to Flora Fairbairn, who sent Inigo my way.

Thank you, Emma Moseley, Hannah Dawson and Nancy Trotter Landry, for being incredible friends. Huge love and thanks to Bill and Sally Lee: I am sorry I had to give up smoking, but I will hang around a pickup truck talking horses and drinking Coke with you any day. Heartfelt thanks to Dave Motion, without whom my computer would never work and I would not be able to write anything.

Thanks to my community on Instagram, who are such an important and enduring part of my daily life. You encourage me and inspire me, and the virtual conversations I have with so many of you have become a part of my creativity and motivation.

Thank you to Charlie Cory Wright and Neil Grundon for wisdom in hard times, and to Juliet Nicolson for some important conversations. Thank you to Tiffany Roy, for support and knowledge and friendship. Thank you to Nick Jenkins, for a beautiful room to write in. Thank you to the Clifford family in Frampton on Severn, especially Rollo and Janie, Charlie and Pete, and Sarah Clifford. I wrote the first chapter of this book at their house, a place where Nell had felt much at home, over five extraordinarily hot days in the summer of 2020. The hypnotic experience of walking alone at dusk in the pounding heat amongst the rosemary bushes and under the fig tree in the garden Nell had loved was a bit like being in a trance. Those days in Frampton on Severn, where I felt that my sister's spirit was beside me, were instrumental in helping me understand what I was trying to do with my words.

Thank you to Caroline Wood for early words of encouragement, to Abigail Bergstrom for a bit in the middle, and thanks, Robert Caskie, here's to the future.

A huge, huge thank-you to the incredible team at Doubleday for their belief in me. I am especially grateful to Susanna Wadeson, who edits like the most meticulous seamstress, unpicking knots here, cutting whole panels of work to replace with new tucks there, adding shots of colour and then stitching the entire thing together, knowing when is the exact moment to put the needle and thread down and stand back to admire the new outfit. Thank you, Alison Barrow, for so much support and care, more than anything, and for really understanding who I am as a writer. Thanks to Helena Gonda, Kate Samano, Ruth Richardson, Dan Prescott, Marianne Issa El-Khoury, Anna Morrison, Richenda Todd, Lorraine Jerram and Lorraine McCann.

Thank you to Laura and Paul Emerson for so much love and support, and thank you to Toti and Alice, Red and Cecil and Peggy for just being you. And *I love you* to my brother Tom and my sisters Emma and Sophy.

I talked to my stepmother, Alexandra Pringle, and my father, Rick Stroud, multiple times a week, sometimes multiple times a day, while I was writing this book. Nell's death shattered so much, but I am profoundly, deeply grateful to you both for your very existence.

Thanks, kids – Jimmy, Dolly, Evangeline, Dash and Lester – for your kindness, love, energy, sweetness, jokes, enthusiasm and the way (some of) you scream really loudly in the kitchen so I know it's time to stop work.

Most of all, my complete love to Pete. You are my light and my dark and I owe you everything.

Clover Stroud is a writer and journalist, writing regularly for the *Sunday Times*, *Guardian* and *Saturday* and *Sunday Telegraph*, among others. Her first book, *The Wild Other*, was shortlisted for the Wainwright Prize. Her critically acclaimed second book, *My Wild and Sleepless Nights: A Mother's Story*, was rated one of the 'best books of the year, 2020' by the *Observer*, *Telegraph* and *Sunday Times*, and was a *Sunday Times* bestseller. She lives in Oxfordshire with her husband and five children.